Memorix N

Memorix

The *Memorix* series consists of easy to use pocket books in a number of different medical and surgical specialities. They contain a vast amount of practical information in very concise form through the extensive use of tables and charts, lists and hundreds of clear line diagrams, often in two colours.

Memorix will give students, junior doctors and some of their senior colleages a handy and comprehensive reference in their pockets.

Other titles in the series include:

Obstetrics
Thomas Rabe

Gynecology
Thomas Rabe

Emergency Medicine
Sönke Müller

Surgery
Jürgen Hußmann and Robert Russell

Physiology
Robert Schmidt, W.D. Willis and L. Reuss

Pediatrics
Dieter Harms and Jochem Scharf

Memorix

Neurology

Peter Berlit

Translated by E.H. Jellinek

CHAPMAN & HALL MEDICAL

London · Glasgow · Weinheim · New York ·
Tokyo · Melbourne · Madras

Published by Chapman & Hall, 2–6 Boundary Row, London SE1 8HN, UK

Chapman & Hall, 2–6 Boundary Row, London SE1 8HN, UK

Blackie Academic & Professional, Wester Cleddens Road, Bishopbriggs, Glasgow G64 2NZ, UK

Chapman & Hall GmbH, Pappelallee 3, 69469 Weinheim, Germany

Chapman & Hall USA, 115 Fifth Avenue, New York NY 10003, USA

Chapman & Hall Japan, ITP-Japan, Kyowa Building, 3F, 2-2-1 Hirakawacho, Chiyoda-ku, Tokyo 102, Japan

Chapman & Hall Australia, 102 Dodds Street, South Melbourne, Victoria 3205, Australia

Chapman & Hall India, R. Seshadri, 32 Second Main Road, CIT East, Madras 600 035, India

English language edition 1996

© 1996 Chapman & Hall

Original German language edition – *Memorix Spezial Neurologie* © 1994 Chapman & Hall GmbH, 69469 Weinheim, Germany.

Typeset in Times by Best-set Typesetter Ltd., Hong Kong
Printed and bound in Hong Kong

ISBN 0 412 56070 4

Apart from any fair dealing for the purposes of research or private study, or criticism or review, as permitted under the UK Copyright Designs and Patents Act, 1988, this publication may not be reproduced, stored, or transmitted, in any form or by any means, without the prior permission in writing of the publishers, or in the case of reprographic reproduction only in accordance with the terms of the licences issued by the Copyright Licensing Agency in the UK, or in accordance with the terms of licences issued by the appropriate Reproduction Rights Organization outside the UK. Enquiries concerning reproduction outside the terms stated here should be sent to the publishers at the London address printed on this page.
  The publisher makes no representation, express or implied, with regard to the accuracy of the information contained in this book and cannot accept any legal responsibility or liability for any errors or omissions that may be made.
  The doses of medicaments have been carefully checked but the author, translator and publishers cannot guarantee correctness, and the reader is advised to refer and re-check by using the manufacturers' instruction leaflets and appropriate pharmacological texts, particularly where new and unfamiliar preparations are concerned.

A catalogue record for this book is available from the British Library

Library of Congress Catalog Card Number: 94-74704

Contents

Preface   xv

Neurological symptoms and syndromes   1

Differential diagnosis of papilloedema   1
Cranial nerves, function, testing and causes of lesions   2
Pupil: reaction to light   4
Abnormal pupil reactions   5
Clinical and pharmacological differentiation of anisocoria   6
Causes of ptosis   7
Horner's syndrome   7
Pseudoptosis   7
Cranial nerve lesions and eye movements   8
Internuclear ophthalmoplegia   9
Eye movements and visual field defects   10
Disorders of taste   12
Facial palsy: Causes   13
Facial palsies at different levels of lesion   14
Hearing tests   15
Causes of deafness and tinnitus   16
Differential diagnosis of common forms of nystagmus   17
Unusual kinds of nystagmus   18
Differential diagnosis of vertigo and giddiness   19
Multiple cranial nerve deficits: differential diagnosis   20
Motor pathways   21
Reflexes   24
Testing muscle strength: grades of power   24
Relation of reflexes to spinal cord segments and peripheral nerves   25
Important limb muscles and their innervation   27
Motor and sensory cortical areas   28
Somatovisceral sensitivity   29
Typical sensory disorders with lesions of different locations   29
Sensory connections   30
Sensory symptoms   31
Anatomy of spine, cord and roots   32
Dermatomes and peripheral sensory nerves   33
Stretching roots and meninges   35
Pyramidal tract signs   36
Pathological reflexes and signs   37
Cerebellar functions   38
Disorders of cerebellar function   39
Cerebellum viewed from above and below   40
Schema of autonomic nervous system   41

MEMORIX NEUROLOGY

Functions of sympathetic and parasympathetic nervous systems	42
Functions of sympathetic nerves and localization of sweating disorders	43
Autonomic function assessment	44
Tests of sweating	45
Bladder function	46
Bladder disorders	46
Neurogenic bladder disorders	47
Neuroanatomy of bladder disorders	48
Neurogenic bladder disorders: causes and treatment	49
Cortex: integrative functions	50
Grades of anosognosia	51
Important neuropsychological disorders	51
Speech: aphasia	52
Higher mental function testing	53
Cognitive differences of the two hemispheres	54
Dysarthrias	55
Central and neuromuscular disorders of respiration	56
Neuromuscular disorders	57
Causes of disorders of consciousness	58
Mental state assessment	59
Mental disorders with an organic basis	60
Brain syndromes	61

Investigative procedures and laboratory diagnosis in neurology 63

Doppler sonography of extracranial arteries supplying the brain	63
Transcranial sonography	64
Identification criteria of intracranial arteries by transcranial Doppler sonography	65
Doppler sonography criteria for degree of carotid stenosis	66
Electroencephalography (EEG)	67
EEG electrode positioning in 10–20 System	68
EEG frequency bands	69
Physical parameters for polygraph recording	69
Variants of normal EEG	70
Stages of sleep in the EEG	71
Brain mapping (EEG cartography)	72
Electromyography (EMG): needle electrode myography	73
EMG patterns: normal, neuropathic, myopathic	73
Needle EMG of important muscles: normal findings	74
Nerve conduction velocity of median nerve	75

CONTENTS

Nerve conduction velocity of tibial nerve	75
Nerve conduction velocity of common peroneal nerve	76
Nerve conduction velocity of sural nerve	76
Nerve conduction velocity of ulnar nerve	77
Normal range of F wave, H reflex and blink reflex	78
Repetitive nerve stimulation electromyography	78
Latency ranges of evoked potentials	79
Visual evoked potentials (VEP) results in different conditions	80
Specific VEP abnormalities: diagnostic significance	80
Auditory evoked potentials (AEP): diagnostic criteria	81
AEP: indication of site of lesion by peak drop-out	81
Indications for use of AEP in diagnosis	82
Auditory pathways – AEP	83
Characteristic AEP changes of some diseases	84
AEP: normal values	85
Somatosensory evoked potentials (SSEP): lead positions and response potentials	86
Siting of leads for somatosensory potentials (SSEP) according to 10–20 scheme	87
Common sites for stimulation and recording in SSEP diagnosis	87
Critical data in SSEP diagnosis in general	88
Assessment criteria in SSEP diagnosis	88
Pathophysiology of SSEP or impulse conduction by underlying disorder	88
Clinical significance of SSEP diagnosis	89
Clinical application of SSEP	89
Dynamic (serial) application of SSEP	89
Common SSEP abnormalities in some clinical conditions	90
Prognostic significance of certain SSEP in severe cerebral disorders	90
SSEP in disorders of the spinal cord	91
Median nerve SSEP at different levels (normal data)	92
Normal data for SSEP from tibial nerve stimulation	93
Normal data for SSEP from trigeminal nerve stimulation	93
Magnetic stimulation: motor evoked potentials (MEP)	94
Magnetic stimulation sites	95
Magnetic stimulation: normal range	96
Indications for lumbar puncture	97
Cerebrospinal fluid (CSF)	97
Common constellations of CSF abnormalities	98
CSF changes in diseases of the nervous system	99
Investigations in cerebrovascular disease	101
Special blood tests	102
Blood clotting	103

MEMORIX NEUROLOGY

Normal skull X-ray	104
Principles of assessment of spinal X-rays	107
Assessment of craniovertebral junction (X-rays)	109
Computerized tomography (CT) of head	110
Hounsfield numbers for tissue density in head CT	110
Density of lesions in CT of head	111
Effect of contrast injection on CT in common brain lesions	111
Calcification in CT of head	111
Anatomy of arteries of the brain	112
Planes of tomographic sections in magnetic resonance imaging (MRI)	113
Relaxation times in MRI related to tissue density	113

Headache 114

Headache: classification	114
Headache: differential diagnosis	116
Differential diagnosis of cluster headache and chronic paroxysmal hemicrania	117
Diagnostic criteria of drug-induced headache	117
Pain localization in neuralgias of face and head	118
Neuralgias and pain in face and head	119
Head and face pain: treatment	120
Migraine treatment	120

Tumours of the nervous system 121

Localization of tumours of the nervous system	121
Treatment and follow-up recommendations for brain tumours in adults	121
Brain tumours: indications for radiotherapy and cytostatic chemotherapy	122
Karnovsky scale for disability grading in neoplastic disease	122
Brain tumours: localization	123
Types of brain herniation with raised intracranial pressure (ICP)	124
Histological classification of tumours of the nervous system	125
Hydrocephalus: differential diagnosis	127
Pituitary tumours: symptoms and signs	128
Diagnosis of pituitary tumours	128
Pituitary hormones: posterior lobe	129
Pituitary hormones: anterior lobe	130
Hypothalamic regulatory hormones	130

CONTENTS

Motor disorders of the central nervous system — 131

- Basal ganglia: functions — 131
- Disease staging of Parkinsonism — 132
- Grading of disability in Parkinsonism — 132
- Idiopathic Parkinsonism: diagnostic criteria — 133
- Apomorphine test — 133
- Parkinsonism: causes — 134
- Glossary of Parkinsonism — 135
- Treatment of Parkinsonism — 136
- Differential diagnosis of tremor — 137
- Mechanisms of tremor production — 138
- Aetiology and treatment of chorea — 139
- Dystonias and dyskinesias — 140
- The myoclonias — 141
- Myoclonia: selective treatment — 142
- Cerebellar degenerations — 143
- Spinocerebellar disorders: genetics of biochemical abnormalities — 144
- Causes of acquired cerebellar defects — 145

Dementia — 146

- Differential diagnosis of dementia — 146
- Diagnosis of Alzheimer type dementia — 147
- Diagnosis of vascular dementia — 148
- Differential diagnosis of cortical and subcortical dementia — 149
- Differential diagnosis of confusional states — 150

Fits and other attacks — 151

- International classification of epileptic attacks — 151
- Classification of age related and non-age related epilepsies and epileptic syndromes — 152
- Common causes of seizures in different age groups — 153
- Acute treatment of epileptic fits — 153
- Epilepsy: first aid and prognosis — 154
- Medication liable to lower central epileptic threshold and cause occasional fits — 155
- Differential diagnosis of seizures — 156
- Choice of anti-epileptic drugs — 157
- Dosage and pharmacology of main antiepileptic drugs — 158
- Antiepileptic drugs: possible reactions, side-effects and overdosage features — 159

ix

MEMORIX NEUROLOGY

Diagnostic of sudden collapse	160
Non-epileptic attacks	162

Inflammatory diseases of the nervous system 163

Diagnosis and treatment of herpes simplex encephalitis	163
Differential diagnosis of viral encephalitis	164
Bacterial meningitis: causative organisms and treatment	165
Brain abscesses: important causative organisms and antibiotics of choice	166
Entry of antibiotics into the CSF	166
Antibiotic treatment in neurology	166
Treatment indications for neurosyphilis	167
Neurosyphilis: diagnostic testing	168
Neurosyphilis: stages and clinical features	169
Stages of HIV infection	170
Neurological complictions in AIDS	171
Stages of AIDS dementia complex	172
Causes of chronic meningitis	172

Cerebrovascular diseases 173

Classification of cerebral ischaemia	173
Risk factors, concomitant diseases and findings which increase risk of cerebral infarction	173
Diagnosis of cerebral infarction	174
Diagnostic value of investigations in cerebral infarction	174
Important collaterals for cerebral blood supply	175
Pattern of CT changes in cerebral infarction	176
Localizing value of clinical pictures	177
Vascular territories in CT	177
Thalamic infarcts	178
Lacunar infarcts	178
Percentage frequencies of arteriosclerotic obstructions in extracranial arteries to the brain and in the Circle of Willis	179
Crossed brain stem syndromes	180
Vascular territories of the three main cerebral arteries	181
Differential diagnosis of stroke	182
Differential diagnosis of cerebral ischaemia	182
Principles of management of cerebral infarction	183
Anticoagulation in acute cerbral infarction	183
Indication for endarterectomy in internal carotid stenosis	184

CONTENTS

Subclavian steal syndrome	185
Scale of deficits in infarction (NIH stroke scale)	186
Scale of independence after cerebrovascular accident (Barthel scale)	187
Anatomy of cerebral venous drainage	188
Symptoms and signs of cerebral venous sinus thrombosis	189
Venous sinus thrombosis: causes and associated disorders	189
Subarachnoid haemorrhage	190
Common sites of cerebral aneurysms	191
Neurological defects from cerebral aneurysms	191
Estimation of age of intracerebral haematoma by MRI through demonstration of methaemoglobin	192
Differential diagnosis of intracerebral haematoma from ischaemia	192
Intracerebral haematoma: frequency and causes in various sites	193
Spontaneous intracranial bleeding: diagnostic procedures	193
Main clinical features of intracerebral haematomas	194

Traumatic lesions of the nervous system   195

Craniocerebral trauma: clinical grading	195
Indications for surgery after open and closed craniocerebral injury	195
Glasgow coma scale	196
Glasgow outcome scale	196
Clinical stages of craniocerebral trauma	197
Cranial nerve damage from trauma	199
The risk of epilepsy after head injuries	200
Differential diagnosis of pseudocoma	201
Criteria of brain death	202
Criteria of brain death in different countries	203

Disorders of the spinal cord   204

Cord transection at different levels: clinical features and orthotic measures	204
Spinal cord syndromes: anatomical patterns	205
Non-traumatic acute transverse cord lesions: differential diagnosis	206
Spinal dysrhaphism	207
Blood supply of spinal cord	207
Types of Arnold – Chiari malformation	208
Synopsis of diseases of the spinal cord	209
Spinal muscular atrophies	209

Polyneuropathies — 210

Causes of polyneuropathy — 210
Diagnostic strategies in polyneuropathy — 210
Aetiology of polyneuritis and polyneuropathy — 211
Toxic polyneuropathies — 212
Pharmacologically induced polyneuropathies — 212
Hereditary polyneuropathies — 213
Hereditary polyneuropathies with metabolic and other defects — 214
Guillain – Barré syndrome: definition — 215
Chronic inflammatory demyelinating neuropathy (CIDP): definition — 215
Diet in phytanic acid storage (Refsum's) disease — 216
Varieties of immunoneuropathy — 216
Features of autonomic involvement in polyneuropathy — 217
Treatment possibilities for polyneuropathy — 218

Peripheral nerve lesions — 219

Areas of referred pain — 219
Syndromes of cervical spinal root compression from intervertebral disc prolapse — 220
Syndromes of lumbosacral spinal root compression from intervertebral disc prolapse — 221
Causes of lumbosacral root disorders — 222
Non-radicular neurological causes of lower limb pain — 222
Classification of peripheral nerve injuries — 223
Differential diagnosis of brachial plexus from cervical root lesions — 223
Brachial plexus lesions — 224
Brachial plexus: root supply (C4–T1) and peripheral distribution — 225
Main features of brachial plexus lesions — 225
Median nerve lesions — 226
Ulnar nerve lesions — 227
Radial nerve lesions — 228
Tibial nerve lesions — 229
Peroneal nerve lesions — 229
Femoral nerve lesions — 230
Sciatic nerve lesions — 230
Obturator nerve lesions — 230
Lateral cutaneous nerve of the thigh lesions — 230
Gluteal nerve lesions — 230
Pudendal nerve lesions — 230
Compartment syndrome — 231
Differential diagnosis of important peripheral nerve lesions — 232

CONTENTS

Muscle diseases 237

Muscle diseases: diagnostic procedures	237
Benign congenital myopathies	237
Congenital diseases of muscle (dystrophies, myotonias, myopathies of metabolic diseases, congenital myopathies; glycogenoses)	238
Mitochondrial myopathies	240
Malignant hyperpyrexia	241
Muscular dystrophies: genetics and natural history	242
Mitochondrial multisystem disorders (myoencephalopathies)	243
Myopathies: metabolic function tests	245
Causes of myoglobinuria	246
Ion channel disorders	246
Grading of myasthenia gravis	247
Motor (neuromuscular) end-plate	247
Tensilon test	248
Myasthenia treatment: anticholinesterases	248
Surgery in myasthenia: practical procedures	248
Differentiating of myasthenic from cholinergic crisis	249
Myasthenia: medications to be avoided and alternatives	250

Multifocal neurological disorders 251

Dyskalaemic periodic paralyses	251
Paraneoplastic neurological disorders	251
Neurological features of endocrine disorders	252
Multiple sclerosis: classification	253
Impairment (Kurtzke) scale in multiple sclerosis	253
Multiple sclerosis – CAMBS scale	254
Multiple sclerosis: typical features	255
Phacomatoses	256
The porphyrias	257
Prohibited medicaments in porphyrias and permissible alternatives	257
Alcoholism: disorders of nervous system and muscle	258
Alcohol withdrawal: principles of management	259
Neurological causes in disorders of swallowing	259
Diagnostic criteria of cranial (temporal) arteritis	260
Laboratory investigations in suspected vasculitis and collagenoses	260
Vasculitis survey	261
Neurological effects of vitamin deficiencies	262
Stages of normal sleep during one night	263
Sleep disorders	264

MEMORIX NEUROLOGY

Pathogenesis of obstructive sleep apnoea — 265
Varieties of sleep apnoea — 265

Therapeutic problems in neurology — 266

Effectiveness profile of neuroleptic drugs — 266
Classification of organically determined cerebral psychosyndromes — 266
Treatment with botulinum toxin — 267
Neurological medication in pregnancy — 268
Options for plasmapheresis treatment in neurology — 269
Options for immunosuppressant treatment in neurology — 269
Immunosuppressant treatment options in neurological diseases — 270

Chromosome anomalies in neurological diseases — 271
Index — 272

Preface

Memorix – Neurology has reached its third edition and has been translated into six languages: apparently it serves its purpose as a companion in the coat pocket. In order to do so the third edition has been completely revised, complemented and brought up to date. I have been assisted in this by R. Diehl (clinical neuropsychology), D. Linden (magnetic stimulation) and E. Möbius (bladder disorders) and wish to record my heartfelt thanks. I have taken up stimuli and suggestions for improvement from the readers and would be grateful for critical comments also on this edition.

Peter Berlit
Essen

MEMORIX NEUROLOGY

Translator's note

While students and practitioners of neurology have a wide choice of excellent English texts from both sides of the Atlantic on principles and practice at all levels, right up to the multivolume Handbook of Clinical Neurology (Vinken, Bruyn, Klawans (eds): Elsevier, Amsterdam) there is a place for a pocket reference book. Inevitably this means a work of lists and tables which feature 'small print' conditions as well as the commoner problems.

I have made minor alterations from the German original to conform with practice in English speaking countries in investigations and treatments, have curtailed and modified overlaps with psychiatry and haematology and have added some English references.

The reader may find some unfamiliar eponyms useful for clinical 'one-upmanship' and, more seriously, common ground for a future European Board examination in neurology. Obviously whenever possible colleagues in the laboratories should be consulted, particularly in the treatment of infections.

E.H. Jellinek
Edinburgh

Acknowledgements

Special thanks to Dr S. Ghattan, University of Washington School of Medicine, Seattle, Washington, USA, for reading the manuscript and suggesting some helpful modifications to the text to bring it in line with current North American practice.

Short contents

Neurological symptoms and syndromes	1
Investigative procedures and laboratory diagnosis in neurology	63
Headache	114
Tumours of the nervous system	121
Motor disorders of the central nervous system	131
Dementia	146
Fits and other attacks	151
Inflammatory diseases of the nervous system	163
Cerebrovascular diseases	173
Traumatic lesions of the nervous system	195
Disorders of the spinal cord	204
Polyneuropathies	210
Peripheral nerve lesions	219
Muscle diseases	237
Multifocal neurological disorders	251
Therapeutic problems in neurology	266
Chromosome anomalies in neurological diseases	271
Index	272

NEUROLOGICAL SYMPTOMS AND SYNDROMES

Differential diagnosis of papilloedema

Congestive (plerencephalic) papilloedema No visual loss	Papillitis Acute loss of vision Pain	Anterior ischaemic optic neuropathy Acute loss of vision No pain
Tumours Haemorrhages Infarction with brain oedema Sinus thrombosis Craniocerebral trauma Faulty CSF circulation High CSF protein (Guillain–Barré syndrome, subarachnoid haemorrhage) Endocrinopathies Metabolic causes Toxic causes	Multiple sclerosis Tuberculosis Guillain–Barré syndrome Bacterial meningitis Sinusitis Inflammations of orbit	Arteriosclerosis (hypertension, diabetes mellitus) Carotid stenosis Vasculitides (cranial arteritis, collagenoses) Haematological disorders (polycythaemia)

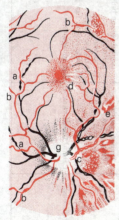
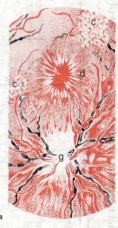

a Arteriovenous nipping
b Splaying of vessels
c Cotton wool spot
d Exudate
e Haemorrhage
f Irregular vessel wall
g Swollen disc/papilloedema

NB Fluorescein angiography to differentiate pseudopapilloedema.

MEMORIX NEUROLOGY

Cranial nerves, function, testing and causes of lesions

Cranial nerve	Function	Testing	Main causes of lesions	Comments
I Olfactory	Smell	Aromatics	Trauma, olfactory groove meningioma, inflammation, viruses, drugs	Complaints of disordered taste
II Optic	Vision	Visual acuity, visual fields, funduscopy	Optic neuritis, papillitis, papilloedema, ischaemic optic neuropathy optic nerve tumour, trauma, Leber's optic atrophy, chiasmal compression (pituitary tumour)	Field defects from optic tract and visual cortex lesions
III Oculomotor	Levator palpebrae, inferior and superior rectus, inferior oblique and sphincter pupillae muscles	Ptosis, eye movements, pupil	Diabetes, posterior communicating artery aneurysm, raised intracranial pressure, tumour, trauma, vascular	Pressure lesions usually affect pupil; differential diagnosis internuclear ophthalmoplegia
IV Trochlear	Superior oblique muscle	Eye movements	Trauma, vascular causes, tumour	Ocular' torticollis' (head tilt)
V Trigeminal	Sensation: face, eye tongue, partly oropharynx Jaw muscles	Sensory: peripheral and central (onion bulb pattern) Jaw deviates to paralysed side Corneal reflex, Jaw jerk	Trigeminal neuralgia and neuropathy, brain stem lesions (vascular and inflammatory) acoustic neuroma, skull-base tumour, trauma	Association with supratentorial lesions
VI Abducens	Lateral rectus muscle	Eye movements	Inflammatory, raised intracranial pressure craniocerebral trauma, multiple sclerosis, parainfectious and vascular causes, congenital	Commonest single eye muscle palsy

NEUROLOGICAL SYMPTOMS AND SYNDROMES

Cranial nerves, function, testing and causes of lesions (continued)

Cranial nerve	Function	Testing	Main causes of lesions	Comments
VII Facial	Facial muscles Tear and salivary glands Stapedius muscle Taste anterior two-thirds of tongue	Miming (eyebrows up, eye closure, baring teeth) Schirmer's test (tear secretion) Stapedius reflex Taste testing	Idiopathic, geniculate herpes, petrous fracture, polyneuritis, borreliosis tumours, Melkersson–Rosenthal syndrome, surgical lesion	Central causes spare upper face Peripheral lesions: Bell's phenomenon
VIII Vestibulo-Cochlear	Hearing Balance	Hearing tests (including Rinne's and Weber's) Tests for nystagmus	Menière's disease, labyrinthitis, petrous fracture, acoustic neuroma, vascular, benign positional vertigo	Vertigo with vertebro-basilar ischaemia
IX Glosso-pharyngeal	Pharynx muscles (swallowing) Sensation back of tongue, pharynx, middle ear Taste posterior one-third tongue Salivation	Taste testing Salivation Gag reflex Pharynx sensitivity	Brain stem vascular disease, neuroma, glomus jugulare tumour, surgical lesions, neuralgia	Single nerve lesion is unusual
X Vagus	Parasympathetic innervation Larynx muscles and sensation Soft palate	Soft palate, voice Larynx examination Autonomic tests	Craniocervical junction anomalies, brain stem vascular disease, bulbar palsies, polio, diphtheria, surgery (thyroid: recurrent laryngeal nerve)	Single nerve lesion is unusual
XI Spinal accessory	Sternomastoid muscle Trapezius muscle (partly)	Head rotation and tilt Shoulder elevation	Skull base lesions, polio, surgery	CVA may be accompanied by ipsilateral accessory palsy
XII Hypoglossal	Tongue muscles	Tongue protrusion Deviation to weak side Look for atrophy Dysarthria	Tumours, vascular disease, basal meningitis	Central pareses recover quickly

Pupil: reaction to light

Schematic diagram of the pupillary light reaction

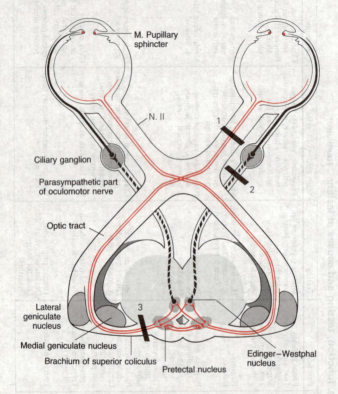

Lesion site 1: normal pupil, visual failure (optic nerve lesion) without direct light reaction
Lesion site 2: paralysis of pupil from third nerve lesion: completely fixed
Lesion site 3: absent light reaction (Argyll Robertson pupil): accommodation–convergence reaction preserved

NEUROLOGICAL SYMPTOMS AND SYNDROMES

Abnormal pupil reactions (right [shown red] is pathological)
(Reproduced from Mummenthaler, M. Neurologies 8th edn; published by Thieme, Stuttgart, 1986.)

	Position at rest (right / left)	Direct light	Light contralateral	Convergence	Peculiarities
Normal	● ●	● ●	● ●	● ●	
Absent afferent pupillary light reflex (vision ↓)	● ●	● ● (no response right)	● ●	● ●	Right eye blind
III nerve lesion (and ciliary ganglion)	● ●	⬤ ●	⬤ ●	⬤ ●	III nerve exernal ocular movement paralysis. Contracts to miotics
Holmes–Adie (myotonic) pupil	● ●	⬤ ●	⬤ ●	⬤ ●	External ocular movements normal, tonic dilation after convergence constriction
Argyll Robertson pupil (lost light reaction)	● ●	● ●	● ●	● ●	Pupils often irregular
Previous optic nerve lesion	● ●	● ●	● ●	● ●	Swinging pen torch test
Atropine effect	⬤ ●	⬤ ●	⬤ ●	⬤ ●	External ocular movements normal, no contraction to miotics

MEMORIX NEUROLOGY

Clinical and pharmacological differentiation of anisocoria

(Reproduced from Berlit, P. *Neurologie in der Praxis*; published by V.C.H., Weinheim, 1988.)

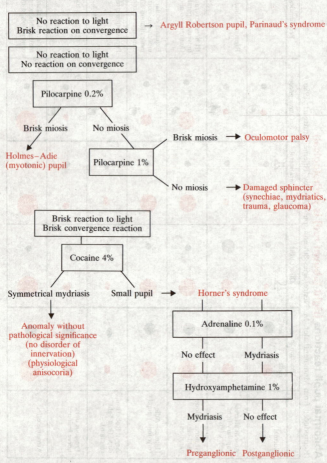

NEUROLOGICAL SYMPTOMS AND SYNDROMES

Causes of ptosis
(Reproduced from Berlit, P. *Klinische Neurologie*; published by V.C.H., Weinheim, 1992.)

Levator palpebrae muscle
- Muscular Dystrophy (ocular, oculopharyngeal, dystrophia myotonica), CPED
- Myasthenia gravis, Botulism
- Oculomotor (III nerve) palsy (diabetes mellitus, tumour, aneurysm, cavernous sinus affections, meningitis, Miller–Fisher syndrome, encephalitis)
- Neurosyphilis (bilateral)
- Muscle compression (orbital space occupying lesions)

Tarsal (Mueller's) muscle

Horner's syndrome
Causes
1. Preganglionic
   First sympathetic neuron (diencephalon – brain stem – 1st thoracic): abnormal sweating same side of body
   (a) Brain stem infarction (Wallenberg's syndrome)
   (b) Syringobulbia
   (c) Tumours
   (d) Inflammation (multiple sclerosis, encephalitis)
   Second sympathetic neuron (spinal cord, cervical sympathetic – superior cervical ganglion): abnormal sweating same side face or upper trunk
   (a) Pancoast tumour
   (b) Aneurysm of aorta
   (c) Neck injuries
2. Postganglionic
   Third sympathetic neurone (superior cervical ganglion – carotid artery – orbit): no disorder of sweating
   (a) Raeder's syndrome, cluster headache, carotidodynia
   (b) Para-sellar tumours
   (c) Carotid artery lesions (dissection, thrombosis, fibromuscular dysplasia, aneurysm)
   (d) Nasopharyngeal tumours

Pseudoptosis
Causes
- Oedema, myxoedema
- Inflammation
- Senile ptosis (slack connective tissue)
- Angioneurotic lid oedema
- Psychogenic: check innervation of orbicularis oculi muscles

MEMORIX NEUROLOGY

Cranial nerve lesions and eye movements

Eye positions in lesions of III, IV and VI nerves
(Modified from Mummenthaler, M. *Neurologie*, 8th edn; published by Thieme, Stuttgart, 1988.)

Right-sided abducens (VI) nerve lesion
looking straight (primary position)

Compensatory head posture (least squint)

Head turned towards side of weak muscle

Maximal squint on looking in direction of action of weak muscle

Right-side trochlear (IV) nerve lesion
looking straight (primary position)

Maximal squint

Head tilt to opposite shoulder. Compensatory posture (Bielschowsky sign)

Compensatory head posture (least squint)

Head tilt to sound side

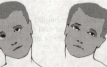

Right-sided oculomotor (III) nerve lesion

Maximal squint position; in severe III nerve lesion the pupil is dilated and fixed

Primary position
No compensatory head posture change as ptosis blocks diplopia

8

NEUROLOGICAL SYMPTOMS AND SYNDROMES

Internuclear ophthalmoplegia

May be a feature of:
multiple sclerosis, brain stem infarction, encephalitis, tumours

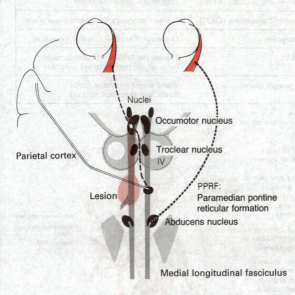

A **lesion of the medial longitudinal fasciculus** (frequently bilateral) between the pontine gaze centres and the III (oculomotor) nucleus region produces a disorder of innervation of the contralateral medial rectus muscle, with intact ipsilateral abducens nerve function. On attempting lateral gaze the adducting eye fails to turn in and the abducting eye may exhibit horizontal nystagmus (dissociated or 'ataxic' nystagmus). The convergence reactions are intact, i.e. the medial rectus functions on convergence.

In the 'one and a half syndrome' internuclear ophthalmoplegia towards the opposite side is combined with a homolateral conjugate horizontal gaze palsy (lesion of the caudal medial longitudinal bundle and of the paramedian pontine reticular formation).

MEMORIX NEUROLOGY

Eye movements and visual field defects

Eye movement production (5 separate systems)

1	Vestibulo-ocular reflex (VOR)	Labyrinth – vestibular nuclei
2	Optokinetic nystagmus (OKN)	Retina – accessory brain stem visual nuclei
3	Convergence	Oculomotor nerve – reticular formation
4	Saccades	Frontal eye fields – reticular formation (vertical and horizontal are separate)
5	Slow pursuit movements	Visual cortex – pontine nuclei – cerebellum (flocculus, vermis)

Localization
Nuclei for eye movements: III and IV   Midbrain
VI   Pons

Visual field defects: localization of lesions

1. *Lesion of optic nerve* (e.g. optic neuritis) Afffecting mainly fibres from the fovea, causing a central scotoma.

2. *Lesion of centre of optic chiasm* produces bi-temporal hemianopia.

3. *Incomplete lesion of right optic tract* causes incongruous homonymous hemianopia in contralateral field of vision.

4. *Incomplete lesion of optic radiation* produces homonymous contralateral upper quadrant field defect.

5. *Complete optic radiation lesion* (and a complete cortical area 17 lesion) causes contralateral homonymous hemianopia.

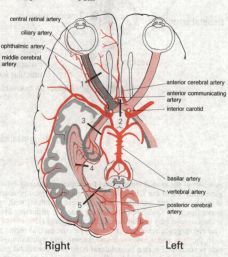

NEUROLOGICAL SYMPTOMS AND SYNDROMES

Eye movements and visual field defects (continued)
Visual field and defect as perceived by

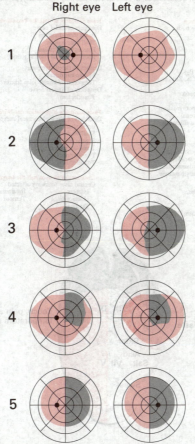

In the charting of visual fields (Bjerrum screen, Friedmann and Goldmann perimetry) the recording is reversed.

MEMORIX NEUROLOGY

Disorders of taste

Pattern of Taste disorders from different causes
(Reproduced after Drester, D. and Conrad, B. Taste disorders following tonsillectomy; published in *Nervenarzt*, 60, 572–5.)

Generalized disorders of taste
Lesions of mucosa or taste buds
  Viral illnesses
  Glossitis, stomatitis
  Sjøgren's syndrome
  Cystic fibrosis
  Radiotherapy
  Vitamin deficiency (A, B_2)
  Electrolyte deficiency (Cu, Zn)
  Toxic
    Alcohol   Tobacco
Hormonal disorders
  Diabetes mellitus   Hypothyroidism
  Pregnancy   Adrenal
                       insufficiency

Drugs
  Penicillamine
  Penicillin   L-dopa
  Griseofulvin   Psychotropics
  Ethambutol   Biguanide
  Metronidazole   Cardamazepine
  Aspirin   Phenylbutazone

Hereditary disorders of taste
  Turner's syndrome
  Riley – Day syndrome
  Pseudohypoparathyroidism

Taste disorders of anterior two-thirds of tongue
Disorders of facial nerve
  Brain stem disorders
  Skull base lesions
  Petrous bone lesions
  Idiopathic facial (Bell's) palsy

Lesions of chorda tympani
  Middle ear disease
  Temporomandibular joint fractures
Disorders of lingual nerve
  Tonsillectomy

Taste disorders of posterior one-third of tongue
Disorders of glossopharyngeal nerve
  Brain stem disorders
  Skull base lesions
  Jugular foramen lesions
  Tonsillar abscess
  Tonsillar tumour
  Tonsillectomy

Disorders of taste of half the tongue (front to back)
Central taste pathways affected
  Infarcts   Inflammation
  Haemorrhage   Tumour
  Trauma

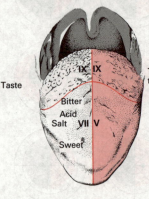

NEUROLOGICAL SYMPTOMS AND SYNDROMES

Facial palsy: causes

(Reproduced after Berlit, P. *Klinische Neurologie*; published by V.C.H., Weinheim, 1992.)

Central type (frontal branch spared, lid closure complete)
- Cerebral infarction
- Intracerebral bleed
- Tumours

Peripheral type (lower motor neuron: Bell's phenomenon, frontal branch involved)
Nuclear with pontine infarction, tumours, haemorrhages
Peripheral (in facial canal, possibly also chorda tympani, nerves to stapedius, petrosus)
Idiopathic (viral)
- Herpes zoster ('geniculate' herpes, Ramsay Hunt syndrome and trigeminal or cervical herpes zoster)
- Otitis media, mastoiditis
- Trauma (basal fractures)
- Tumours (parotid, neurinoma)
- Iatrogenic (after neuroma surgery)
- Nuclear aplasia of Möbius

Mainly bilateral
Polyneuritis cranialis
- Guillain–Barré syndrome
- Tick-borne radiculopathy

Meningitis
- Tuberculous
- Syphilitic

Granulomas
- Melkersson–Rosenthal syndrome
- Sarcoidosis
- Wegener's granulomatosis

Tetanus

Meningeal infiltration
- Carcinomatous
- Leukaemic

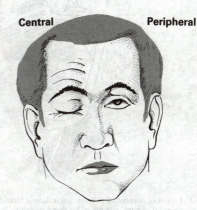

Central   Peripheral

MEMORIX NEUROLOGY

Facial palsies at different levels of lesion

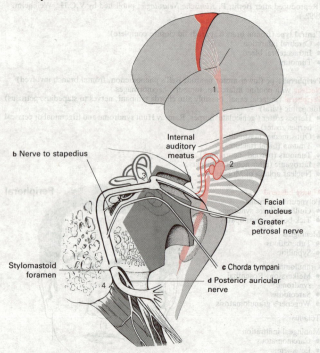

1. Lesion of corticobulbar tract: contralateral facial weakness of central type: good lid closure, sparing of forehead mobility.
2. Nuclear brain stem lesion: ipsilateral facial paralysis of peripheral type without accompaniments.
3. Peripheral lesion in facial canal: ipsilateral weakness of peripheral type, with Bell's phenomenon, and according to site:
   (a) Disordered lacrimation (abnormal Schirmer test)
   (b) Hyperacusis (absent stapedius reflex)
   (c) Disordered taste anterior two-thirds of tongue
   (d) Pain, and complaint of abnormal feeling in front of ear.
4. Extracranial lesion of motor part of VII nerve, or its branches.

NEUROLOGICAL SYMPTOMS AND SYNDROMES

Hearing tests
Weber's and Rinne's tests for conductive or perceptive deafness

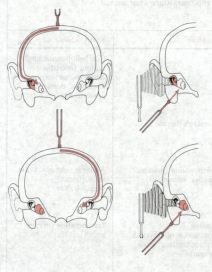

Conductive hearing loss right ear

Perceptive hearing loss right ear

A Weber's test

Application of tuning fork to vertex: patient indicates whether sound is heard in centre of head or lateralized to one ear

Conductive (middle ear) deafness
   Lateralization to affected ear

Perceptive (inner ear) deafness
   Lateralization to unaffected (better) ear

B Rinne's test

Tuning fork is first applied to mastoid process (bone conduction) and when sound no longer perceived held next to external meatus (air conduction)

Assessment:
Rinne's test *normal* (= positive)
   Air conduction perceived about twice as long as bone conduction (30 s longer)

Rinne's test *abnormal* (= negative)
   Air conduction briefer than bone conduction

Conductive (middle ear) deafness
   Rinne's test abnormal (negative)

Perceptive (inner ear or nerve) deafness
   Rinne's test normal (positive)

MEMORIX NEUROLOGY

Causes of deafness and tinnitus

Conductive deafness Weber's test referred to affected ear Rinne's test abnormal	Perceptive deafness Weber's test referred to good ear; Rinne's test normal	
Middle ear	Cochlear	Retrocochlear
Wax Foreign body		Cerebellopontine angle tumour (acoustic neuroma, meningioma, aneurysm, dermoid, epidermoid)
Inflammation (otitis, mastoiditis, cholesteatoma)	Ménière's disease	
Trauma (rupture of drum, dislocation of ossicles)	Inflammation (mumps, measles, meningitis)	Multiple sclerosis, brain stem glioma, syringobulbia
Tumour (glomus jugulare, carcinoma)	Trauma (concussion of labyrinth, petrous fracture, noise trauma)	Inflammation (herpes zoster)
Otosclerosis	Tumour (glomus jugulare, carcinoma)	Brain stem infarction
	Toxic (streptomycin, cisplatinum, aminoglycosides)	
	Congenital (maternal rubella)	
	Vasculitis (Cogan's syndrome) Internal auditory artery occlusion	

NEUROLOGICAL SYMPTOMS AND SYNDROMES

Differential diagnosis of common forms of nystagmus

(Reproduced after Berlit, P. (1988) *Neurologie in der Praxis*, V.C.H., Weinheim)

Terminology	Vertigo	Nystagmus	Associated symptoms
Benign positional vertigo	Paroxysmal rotatory vertigo with change of position (accommodates)	Lasts seconds with change of position (accommodates) towards subjacent ear	None
Ménière's disease	Recurrent attacks of rotatory vertigo	Paroxysmal directional spontaneous nystagmus towards affected ear	Tinnitus, deafness
Vestibular neuropathy	Persistent rotatory vertigo	Directional spontaneous nystagmus toward opposite side	Nausea, vomiting
Vertebro-basilar ischaemia	Variable rotatory vertigo or unsteadiness	Variable directional spontaneous nystagmus, often rotational component	Brain stem symptoms and signs
Labyrinthine apoplexy	Persistent rotatory vertigo	Directional spontaneous nystagmus towards opposite side	Deafness
Congenital nystagmus	None	Pendular, variable direction, enhanced by fixation	None
Ataxic (dissociated) nystagmus	None	Gaze nystagmus, worse in abducting eye, fatigues; poor adduction	Oscillopsia, internuclear ophthalmoplegia
Vertical nystagmus (cerebellar dissociated)	Slight, instability	Up- or down-beat spontaneous or gaze nystagmus	Ataxia, dysarthria
Cerebello-pontine angle lesion	Slight, non-specific	(Early) Directional, spontaneous nystagmus, (advanced) Gaze-evoked nystagmus	Deafness, tinnitus, VII paresis, reduced ophthalmic nerve sensation

Unusual kinds of nystagmus
(Reproduced after Berlit, P. *Neurologie in der Praxis*; published by V.C.H., Weinheim, 1988.)

Terminology	Description	Cause
Muscle paresis nystagmus	Irregular nystagmus of healthy eye in direction of action of paretic muscle	Eye muscle paresis
Gaze paresis Nystagmus	Slow nystagmus on gaze away from (cortical), or towards (pontine), side of lesion	Recovery stage of conjugate deviation
Alternating nystagmus	Spontaneous horizontal nystagmus with periodic alteration of direction	Brain stem lesions
See-saw nystagmus	Vertical alternating see-sawing of eyes with rotatory component	Diencephalic lesions
Nystagmus retractory with clonus of convergence	Rhythmic retraction of eyeballs with convergent jerking	Parinaud's syndrome (upward gaze palsy, poor convergence, abnormal pupils)
Rebound nystagmus	Fatiguable gaze nystagmus with corrective jerks after return to midposition	Cerebellar lesions
Opsoclonus	Rapid repetitive eye conjugate movements in different directions increased by fixation	Cerebellar lesions, particularly paraneoplastic
Ocular Bobbing	Rapid downward jerks with slower return movement (with horizontal gaze palsy)	Pontine lesions
Myoclonic Nystagmus	Rotatory twitches of one eye in line of action of superior oblique muscle	Idiopathic myokymia (myoclonicity) of superior oblique muscle
Cervical Nystagmus	Rapidly fading horizontal nystagmus on trunk rotation with head fixed (in opposite direction)	Disorder of proprioception in degenerative changes of cervical spine

NEUROLOGICAL SYMPTOMS AND SYNDROMES

Differential diagnosis of vertigo and dizziness

	Peripheral labyrinthine	Central vestibular
Positional dizziness		
Latency	Up to 20 s	None
Nystagmus duration	Up to 30 s	Longer than 30 s
Complaint of vertigo	Strong, directional	Not severe, non-directional
Direction of nystagmus	Towards subjacent ear	Variable
Critical head position	Often unique	Usually more than one position
Clinical conditions	Benign positional vertigo	Acoustic neuroma: late feature
	Alcoholic positional vertigo	Vertebrobasilar ischaemia
	Perilymph fistula	Multiple sclerosis
Persistent vertigo and dizziness		
Nystagmus	Horizontal rotatory	Variable: may be up- or down-beat
Associated symptoms	Sometimes deafness, tinnitus	Ocular tilt reaction
Clinical conditions	Ménière's disease	Staggering, oscillopsia, other focal signs: cerebellar or pontomedullary stem lesion – ischaemia, tumour, inflammation, malformation, toxic
	Acute labyrinthine lesion	
	Vestibular neuronitis (without deafness)	
	Acoustic neuroma: early stages	

Causes of vertigo and giddiness

Vestibular			Non-vestibular		
Labyrinth	Vestibular nerve	Central vestibular	Cardiovascular	Psychogenic	Other
Ménière's disease (hydrops of endolymph)	Cerebellopontine angle tumour	Vertebrobasilar ischaemia	Blood pressure changes	Fear of height	Somatosensory cervical vertigo (ageing)
Benign positional vertigo	Vestibular neuronitis	Syringobulbia	Heart rhythm changes	Psychoses	Blood disease: anaemia, leukaemia etc.
Concussion and apoplexy of labyrinth		Temporal lobe epilepsy	Cardiac failure	Phobic episodic dizziness	Hormonal (thyroid disease)
Inflammations Otitis, labyrinthitis, mastoiditis		Multiple sclerosis	Carotid sinus syndrome		Visual (diplopia, sight disorders, superior oblique muscle myokymia)
Toxic: streptomycin, quinine, aminoglycosides, frusemide		Brainstem tumours	Drugs: antihypertensives, beta-blockers, vasodilators, diuretics		
		Toxic (alcohol, carbon monoxide, phenytoin opiates)			
		Cerebellar lesions			

MEMORIX NEUROLOGY

Multiple cranial nerve deficits: differential diagnosis
(Reproduced from Berlit, P. *Neurologie in der Praxis*; published by V.C.H. Weinheim, 1988.)

Affected cranial nerves	Other symptoms	Designation
I, II	Frontal lobe symptoms	Syndrome of anterior cranial fossa
III, IV, V_1, VI	Headache	Superior orbital fissure syndrome
III, IV, V_1, VI	Proptosis Chemosis	Cavernous sinus syndrome
II, III, IV, V_1, VI	–	Orbital apex syndrome
V, VI	–	Petrous apex syndrome (Gradenigo)
VIII, V_1, V_2, VII, VI	Progressing to homolateral ataxia	Cerebellopontine angle syndrome
IX, X, XI	–	Jugular foramen syndrome (Vernet)
IX, X, XI, XII	–	Syndrome of craniocervical junction (Collet–Siccard)
IX, X, XI, XII	Cervical sympathetic	Retropharyngeal syndrome (Villaret)
V–XII	–	Skull base syndrome (Garcin)

Bilateral and variable multiple cranial nerve deficits

With meningitic symptoms and signs	Basal meningitis (Tuberculosis)
With or without areflexia, papilloedema	Carcinomatous or leukaemic meningitis
With pain	Diabetes mellitus Tick-borne radiculopathy
Without pain	Polyneuritis cranialis, paraproteinaemia (Bing–Neel syndrome), diabetes mellitus, vasculitides (polyarteritis nodosa, Cogan's syndrome, Wegener's granulomatosis), sarcoidosis

NEUROLOGICAL SYMPTOMS AND SYNDROMES

Motor pathways
Motor pathways: schematic survey

(Reproduced after Mummenthaler, M. *Neurologie*; published by Thieme, Stuttgart, 1986, p. 99.)

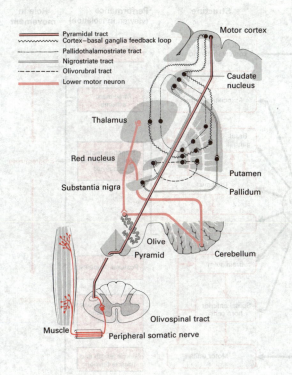

MEMORIX NEUROLOGY

Motor system
(Reproduced after Birnbaumer, N. and Schmidt, R.F. *Biologische Psychologie*; published by Springer, Berlin, 1991.)

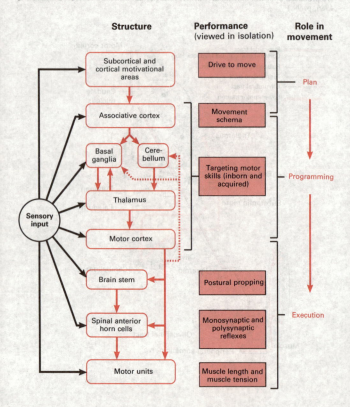

NEUROLOGICAL SYMPTOMS AND SYNDROMES

Motor system (continued)

	Functional anatomy and commentary
Motor unit	Motor neuron in brain stem and spinal cord and innervated muscle fibres. Size from a few muscle fibres in external ocular muscles up to 500–1000 fibres in muscles of the back
Anterior horn of spinal cord	Part of the grey matter contains the interneurons and motor neurons of numerous mono- and polysynaptic motor reflex arcs. Spinal reflexes constitute basis of postural and movement programmes
Brain stem motor centres	From caudal to rostral: 1. medullary portion of reticular formation. 2. motor portions of vestibular nuclei. 3. pontine reticular formation. 4. red nucleus. Main functions of centres: 1. control of posture. 2. coordination with aimed movement. 3. regulation of muscle tone
Motor cortex	1. precentral gyrus (area 4). 2. area 6 with supplementary motor area (SMA) and premotor cortex (PMC): origin of pyramidal tracts (corticospinal tracts). Main function: aimed movement programming (area 4 direction of fine movement, area 6 participation in movement planning)
Motor thalamus	Ventrolateral nucleus (VL) connects cerebellum and basal ganglia with the motor cortex. Main function is integration of sensory and motor inputs
Cerebellum	1. vermis: control of postural propping mechanisms. Pars intermedia: coordination of postural propping with aimed movements. 3. hemispheres: control of fast (acquired, ballistic) aimed movements. Additionally 1 and 2: participation in eye movement control
Basal ganglia	Corpus striatum (putamen and caudate nucleus), globus pallidus, substantia nigra. Main function: elaboration of movement programmes (generation of temporal and spatial pattern of impulses to control amplitude, direction, speed and force of a movement)

Reflexes
Muscle stretch reflexes, cutaneous and other reflexes, their peripheral nerves and spinal roots

Reflex	Peripheral Nerve	Spinal root(s)
Muscle stretch reflex		
Biceps jerk	Musculocutaneous	(C5), C6
Supinator (brachioradialis) jerk	Radial	(C5), C6
Triceps jerk	Radial	C7, (C8)
Finger flexion jerk	Median and ulnar	(C7), C8
Adductor jerk	Obturator	(L2), L3
Knee (quadriceps) jerk	Femoral	L3, L4
Hamstring (semitendinosus) jerk	Sciatic	S1
Tibialis posterior reflex	Tibial	L5
Ankle (calf muscle) jerk	Tibial	S1, S2
Cutaneous and other reflexes		
Superficial abdominal reflexes	Intercostal	T5–T12
Cremasteric reflex	Genitofemoral	L1–2
Anal reflex	Pudendal	S3–S4
Bulbocavernosus reflex	Pudendal	S3–S4

Testing muscle strength: grades of power
(Reproduced from *Aids to the Examination of Peripheral Nerve Lesion*; published by Bailliere Tindall, London, 1986.)

Grade	Definition
0	No muscle contraction visible
1	Barely visible muscle contraction
2	Active movement of part of limb with gravity eliminated
3	Active movement of part of limb against gravity
4–	Active movement against slight resistance
4	Active movement against moderate resistance
4+	Active movement against strong resistance
5	Normal power

NEUROLOGICAL SYMPTOMS AND SYNDROMES

Relation of Reflexes to Spinal Cord Segments and Peripheral Nerves

(Reproduced from Mumenthaler, M. Topographical diagnosis of peripheral nerve lesions, in *Handbook of Clinical Neurology*, vol.2, (eds Vinken, P. and Bruyn, G.), Elsevier, New York, 1969.)

Reflex	Site and mode of elicitation	Response	Muscle(s)	Peripheral nerve(s)	Cord segment(s)
Scapulohumeral reflex	Tap on lower end of medial border of scapula	Adduction and lateral rotation of dependent arm	Infraspinatus and teres minor	Suprascapular (axillary)	C4–C6
Biceps jerk	Tap on tendon of biceps brachii	Flexion at elbow	Biceps brachii	Musulocutaneous	C5, C6
Supinator jerk (also called radial reflex)	Tap on distal end of radius	Flexion at elbow	Brachioradialis (+ biceps brachii and brachialis)	Radial (Musculocutaneous)	C5, C6
Triceps jerk	Tap on tendon of triceps brachii above olecranon, with elbow flexed	Extension at elbow	Triceps brachii	Radial	C7, C8
Thumb reflex	Tap on tendon of flexor pollicis longus in distal third of forearm	Flexion of terminal phalanx of thumb	Flexor pollicis longus	Median	C6–C8
Extensor finger and hand jerk	Tap on posterior aspect of wrist just proximal to radiocarpal joint	Extension of hand and fingers (inconstant)	Extensors of hand and fingers	Radial	C6–C8
Flexor finger jerk	Tap on examiner's thumb placed on palm of hand; sharp tap on tips of flexed fingers (Trömner's sign)	Flexion of fingers	Flexor digitorum superficialis (and profundus)	Median	C7, C8 (T1)
Epigastric reflex (exteroceptive)	Brisk stroking of skin downwards from nipple in mamillary line	Retraction of epigastrium	Transversus abdominis	Intercostal	T5, T6
Abdominal skin reflex (exteroceptive)	Brisk stroking of skin of abdominal wall in lateromedial direction	Shift of skin of abdomen and displacement of umbilicus	Muscles of abdominal wall	Intercostal, hypogastric and ilioinguinal	T7, T12

Relation of reflexes to spinal cord segments and peripheral nerves (continued)

Reflex	Site and mode of elicitation	Response	Muscle(s)	Peripheral nerve(s)	Cord segment(s)
Cremasteric reflex (exteroceptive)	Stroking skin on medial aspect of thigh (pinching adductor muscles)	Elevation of testis	Cremaster	Genital branch of genitofemoral	L2, L3
Adductor reflex	Tap on medial condyle of femur	Adduction of leg	Adductors of thigh	Obturator	L2, L3, L4
Knee jerk	Tap on tendon of quadriceps femoris below patella	Extension at knee	Quadriceps femoris	Femoral	(L2), L3, L4
Gluteal reflex (exteroceptive)	Stroking skin over gluteal region	Tightening of buttock (inconstant)	Gluteus medius and gluteus maximus	Superior and inferior gluteal	L4, L5, S1
Posterior tibial reflex	Tap on tendon of tibialis posterior behind medial malleolus	Supination of foot (inconstant)	Tibialis posterior	Tibial	L5
Semimembranosus and semitendinosus reflex	Tap on medial hamstring tendons (patient prone and knee slightly flexed)	Contraction of semimembranosus and semitendinosus	Semimembranosus and semitendinosus	Sciatic	S1
Biceps femoris reflex	Tap on lateral hamstring tendon (patient prone and knee slightly flexed)	Contraction of biceps femoris	Biceps femoris	Sciatic	S1, S2
Ankle jerk	Tap on Achilles tendon	Plantar flexion of foot	Triceps surae (and other flexors of foot)	Tibial	S1, S2
Bulbocavernosus reflex (exteroceptive)	Gentle squeezing of glans penis or pinching of skin of dorsum of penis	Contraction of the bulbocavernosus muscle, palpable at root of penis	Bulbocavernosus	Pudendal	S3, S4
Anal reflex (exteroceptive)	Scratch or prick of perianal skin (patient lying on side)	Visible contraction of anus	Sphincter ani externus	Pudendal	S5

NEUROLOGICAL SYMPTOMS AND SYNDROMES

Important muscles of the upper limb and their innervation

(Reproduced from Stöhr, M. and Riffel, B. Nerven and *Nervenwurzelläsionen*; published by V.C.H., Weinheim, 1988.)

Muscle	Myotome	Nerve(s)	Test
Supraspinatus and infraspinatus	C4–C6	Suprascapular	External rotation of shoulder
Serratus anterior	C5–C7	Long thoracic (Bell's)	Forward extension of arm
Pectoralis major	C5–D1	Pectoralis	Compression of hands in front of chest
Deltoid	C5–C6	Axillary	Abduction of shoulder
Biceps and brachialis	C5–C6	Musculocutaneous	Elbow flexion in supination
Brachioradialis	C5–C6	Radial	Elbow flexion in midpronation
Triceps	C6–C8	Radial	Elbow extension
Extensor carpi radialis and ulnaris	C6–C8	Radial	Wrist extension
Extensor digitorum	C7–C8	Radial	Finger extension at metacarpophalangeal joint
Extensor and abductor pollicis longus	C7–C8	Radial	Thumb extension and abduction
Pronator teres	C6–C7	Median	Pronation with elbow flexed
Flexor carpi radialis	C6–C7	Median	Wrist flexion (radial direction)
Flexor digitorum sublimis	C7–C8	Median	Finger flexion at proximal interphalangeal joint
Flexor pollicis and profundus of digitorum II and III	C7–C8	Median	Terminal joint flexion of thumb and digitorum II and III
Abductor pollicis brevis	C7–C8	Median	Thumb abduction at 90° from plane of palm
Opponens pollicis	C7–T1	Median	Opposition of thumb towards 5th finger
Flexor carpi ulnaris	C7–T1	Ulnar	Wrist flexion (ulnar direction)
Flexor digitorum profundus IV and V	C7–T1	Ulnar	Terminal joint flexion of digits IV and V
Interossei	C8–T1	Ulnar	Finger spreading and adduction
Adductor pollicis	C8–T1	Ulnar	Thumb adduction (Froment's sign)
Hypothenar (abductor, opponens and flexor brevis of little finger)	C8–T1	Ulnar	Proximal finger movements of little finger
Lumbricals	C7–T1	Median (digits I and II) Ulnar (digits III and IV)	Finger flexion at MCP joints and extension at interphalangeal joints

Muscles of the lower limb

Iliopsoas	L1–L4	Femoral	Hip flexion
Quadruceps femoris	L2–L4	Femoral	Knee extension
Adductors and gracilis	L2–L4	Obturator	Hip adduction
Gluteus medius and minimus	L4–S1	Superior gluteal	Hip abduction
Gluteus maximus	L5–S2	Inferior gluteal	Hip extension
Hamstrings	L5–S2	Sciatic	Knee flexion
Tibialis anterior	L4–5	Common peroneal	Ankle dorsiflexion
Extensor digitorum and extensor hallucis longus	L5–S1	Common peroneal	Dorsiflexion of toes
Peronei	L5–S1	Common peroneal	Ankle eversion
Calf	S1–S2	Tibial	Ankle plantar flexion

Motor and sensory cortical areas
Somatotopic arrangement of primary motor and sensory cortical areas
(Reproduced after Penfield, W. and Rasmussen A.T. *The cerebral cortex of man: a clinical study of localization of function*; published by Macmillan, New York, 1950.)

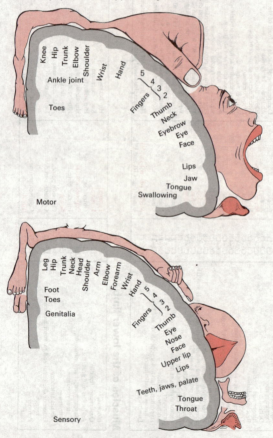

Somatovisceral sensitivity

Types of somatovisceral sensitivity, localization and basic somatovisceral sensors (Reproduced after Birnbaumaer, N. and Schmidt, R.F. *Biologische Psychologie*; published by Springer, Berlin, 1991.)

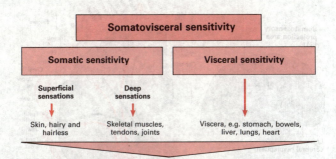

Type of sensor	Examples of relevant stimuli
Mechanical sensor	Pressure, touch, vibration, tension, stretch
Thermal sensor	Cooling, heating
Chemical sensor	Metabolites, pH, pCO_2, pO_2, glucose
Nociceptive sensor	Tissue damage, heat, compression

Typical sensory disorders with lesions of different locations

	Touch	Pain	Temperature	Vibration	Position sense	Symptoms of irritation
Sensory cortex	↓	↓	↓	(↓)	↓↓	Paraesthesiae
Thalamus	↓	↓	↓	↓↓	↓↓	Hyperpathia
Brain stem	↓	↓↓	↓↓	↓	↓	Hyperpathia
Spinothalamic tracts	(↓)	↓↓	↓↓	No abnormality	No abnormality	(Cold) thermal paraesthesiae
Posterior columns	↓↓	No abnormality	No abnormality	↓↓	↓	Paraesthesiae, hyperpathia
Posterior roots	↑ or ↓	↑ or ↓↓	↓↓	↓	↓	Segmental pains
Peripheral nerve	↓↓	↓	↓	↓	↓	Paraesthesiae, causalgia

MEMORIX NEUROLOGY

Sensory connections and important staging points

(Reproduced after Schmidt, R.F. *Medizinische Biologie des Menschen*; published by Piper, Munich, 1983.)

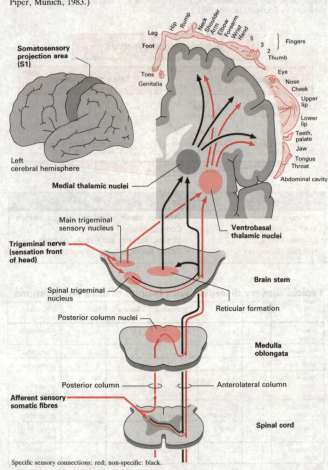

Specific sensory connections: red; non-specific: black.

NEUROLOGICAL SYMPTOMS AND SYNDROMES

Sensory symptoms

(Reproduced after Schmidt, R.F. *Medizinische Biologie des Menschen*; published by Piper, Munich, 1983.)

	Symptoms	Site of lesion	Diseases (Examples)	Treatment
Hyperpathia	Delayed burning pain in hyperaesthetic area, outlasts the stimulus	Thalamus Posterior columns Peripheral nerves Nerve root	Cerebral infarction Spinal cord ischaemia Incomplete nerve injuries Incomplete nerve compression	Carbamazepine Phenytoin Amitriptyline
Paraesthesiae	Tingling Pins and needles Numbness	Sensory cortex Posterior columns Peripheral nerves	Sensory Jacksonian epilepsy B_{12} deficiency Polyneuropathy Root or nerve compression	Carbamazepine Phenytoin Major tranquilizers and neuroleptics TENS
Dysaesthesiae	Altered perception of sensory stimuli	Spinothalamic tracts Nerve roots Peripheral nerves	Myelopathies Intervertebral disc prolapse Nerve compression Polyneuropathy	Amitriptyline Major tranquilizers and neuroleptics TENS
Causalgia	Episodic burning pain, triggered by touch	Peripheral nerve	Incomplete nerve lesions	Sympathetic block Butyrophenones Sympathectomy Major tranquilizers and neuroleptics
Neuralgia	Brief shooting pains along nerve territory	Peripheral nerve	Trigeminal neuralgia Herpes zoster	Carbamazepine Phenytoin
Anaesthesia dolorosa	Causalgic pain in anaesthetic territory	Peripheral nerve	Nerve transection, severe nerve lesions (especially trigeminal)	Major tranquilizers and neuroleptics
Phantom pain	Persistant or episodic pain in non-existent limb	CNS	May follow limb amputation, occasionally after severe brachial plexus lesion	Cordotomy Posterior rhizotomies
Segmental pain	Pain in single dermatome, with hyperaesthesia, worse with stretch or raised intraspinal pressure	Nerve root	Prolapsed intervertebral disc Herpes zoster	Non-steroidal anti-inflammatory agents Nerve blockade Disc surgery

MEMORIX NEUROLOGY

Anatomical levels of spine, cord and roots

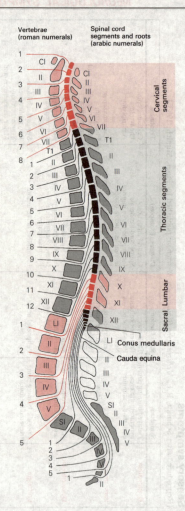

NEUROLOGICAL SYMPTOMS AND SYNDROMES

Dermatomes and peripheral sensory nerves

1. Trigeminal nerve
2. Greater auricular nerve
3. Anterior cutaneous nerve of neck
4. Supraclavicular nerve
5. Intercostal nerve (anterior branch)
6. Lateral cutaneous nerve of arm
7. Medial cutaneous nerve of arm
8. Intercostal nerve (lateral branch)
9. Cutaneous nerve of forearm (posterior branch)
10. Intercostal nerve (anterior branch)
11. Medial cutaneous nerve of forearm
12. Lateral cutaneous nerve of forearm
13. Radial nerve (superficial branch)
14. Median nerve (palmar branch)
15. Median nerve
16. Ulnar nerve
17. Ulnar nerve (palmar branch)
18. Iliohypogastric nerve (lateral branch)
19. Ilioinguinal nerve
20. Iliohypogastric nerve (anterior branch)
21. Genitofemoral nerve
22. Lateral cutaneous nerve of thigh
23. Femoral nerve (anterior cutaneous branches)
24. Obturator nerve
25. Lateral cutaneous nerve of calf of leg
26. Saphenous nerve
27. Superficial peroneal nerve
28. Sural nerve
29. Deep peroneal nerve
30. Tibial nerve

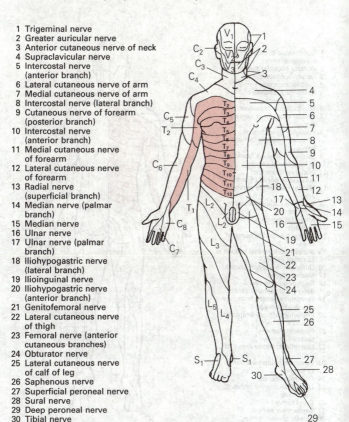

Anterior view of segmental and peripheral sensory innervation
(Modified from Hansen and Schlack. *Segmentale innervation*; published by Thieme, Stuttgart, 1962.)
(also *Aids to the examination of the peripheral nervous system*; published by Baillière Tindall, London, 1980.)

Dermatomes and peripheral sensory nerves (continued)

1. Ophthalmic division of trigeminal nerve
2. Greater occipital nerve
3. Lesser occipital nerve
4. Greater auricular nerve
5. Posterior branches of cervical nerves
6. Supraclavicular nerves
7. Lateral cutaneous nerve of arm
8. Posterior branches of cervical, thoracic, lumbar nerves
9. Lateral cutaneous branches of intercostal nerves
10. Posterior branch of cutaneous nerve of arm
11. Medial cutaneous nerve of arm
12. Posterior cutaneous nerve of forearm
13. Medial cutaneous nerve of forearm
14. Lateral cutaneous nerve of forearm
15. Superficial terminal branch of radial nerve
16. Ulnar nerve (dorsal branch)
17. Median nerve
18. Iliohypogastric nerve (lateral cutaneous branch)
19. Posterior primary branches of lumbar nerves
20. Posterior primary branches of sacral nerves
21. Posterior femoral cutaneous nerve
22. Lateral cutaneous nerve of thigh
23. Posterior cutaneous nerve of thigh
24. Obturator nerve
25. Lateral cutaneous nerve of calf of leg
26. Sural nerve
27. Saphenous nerve
28. Lateral plantar nerve
29. Medial plantar nerve

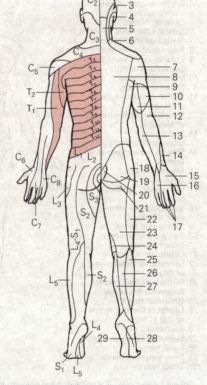

Posterior view of segmental and peripheral sensory innervation
(Modified from Hansen and Schlack. *Segmentale innervation*; published by Thieme, Stuttgart, 1962.)
(also *Aids to the examination of the peripheral nervous system*; published by Baillière Tindall, London, 1980.)

NEUROLOGICAL SYMPTOMS AND SYNDROMES

Stretching roots and meninges
Spinal root and meningeal stretch signs (with root lesions and meningism)

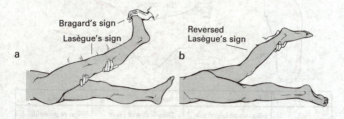

Terminology	Technique	Response	Significance
1. Lasègue	Passive hip flexion with knee straight (patient supine)	Radicular pain	Root compression L4–S1 or meningismus if positive on both sides
2. Reversed Lasègue	Passive hip extension (patient prone)	Radicular pain	Root compression L1–L4
3. Crossed Lasègue	As in Lasègue's test	Pain on opposite side	Marked bilateral root compression
4. Bragard	As in Lasègue's test with additional dorsiflexion of foot	Increased radicular pain	As for Lasègue's, but consider Homan's sign for DVT
5. Kernig	As in Lasègue's test	Knee flexion	Meningismus
6. Brudzinski	Passive flexion of neck	Flexion of both knees	Meningismus

MEMORIX NEUROLOGY

Pyramidal tract signs

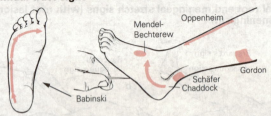

Eponym	Manoeuvre	Response	Significance
Babinski	Scratching lateral side of sole up and medially	Dorsiflexion of great toe and fanning of others	Sign of pyramidal tract lesion
Sicard	Nil	Spontaneous appearance of Babinski sign	Gross pyramidal tract lesion
Brissaud	As for Babinski	Babinski sign plus contraction of tensor fasciae latae muscle	If absent consider possible feigned response
Chaddock	Scratching lateral border of foot upwards below and around lateral malleolus	As for Babinski	As for Babinski
Scherzi	Scratching dorsum of foot around medial malleolus	As for Babinski	As for Babinski
Oppenheim	Forceful downward stroking of shin bone	As for Babinski	As for Babinski
Gordon	Squeezing middle of calf muscles	As for Babinski	As for Babinski
Schäfer	Squeezing distal part of calf muscles	As for Babinski	As for Babinski
Strümpell	Patient flexes knee against examiner's opposing hand	As for Babinski	As for Babinski
Mendel–Bechterew	Percussion of dorsum of foot	Plantar flexion of toes	Exaggerated tendon jerk
Monakow	Stroking lateral border of foot	Elevation of lateral border of foot	As for Babinski
Wartenberg	Flexion of ends of fingers 2–5 against resistance	Thumb flexion and adduction	Pyramidal tract lesion

NEUROLOGICAL SYMPTOMS AND SYNDROMES

Pathological reflexes and signs

Terminology	Manoeuvre	Significance
Glabellar tap, orbicularis oculi or blink reflex	Repeated tapping of glabella	Increased, or fails to fade, with extrapyramidal or supranuclear disorder
Snout or pout reflex (orbicularis oris reflex)	Percussing lips leads to pouting	Elicited with diffuse brain damage
Sucking reflex	Stroking mouth produces sucking	Elicited with severe diffuse brain damage
Grasp reflex	Stroking palm with a finger or an object causes grasping	Elicited with diffuse brain damage
'Magnet' reaction	Hands or head follow objects which are brought close	Elicited with severe diffuse brain damage
'Gegenhalten'	Patient tenses muscles which the examiner tries to stretch	May occur with frontal lobe and basal ganglia lesions
Palmomental reflex	Forceful stroking of palm leads to homolateral chin muscle contraction	Diffuse brain damage
Persistent clonus (jaw, finger, patella, ankle)	Sudden stretching of muscle leads to involuntary repetitive jerking	Pyramidal tract lesion

Cerebellar functions
(Reproduced after Schmidt, R.F. *Memorix Spezial Physiologie*; published by V.C.H., Weinheim, 1992.)
Cerebellar afferent and efferent pathways
1. Median portions of cerebellum (vermis, flocculonodular lobe and pars intermedia)
   (a) Afferents from somatosensory, vestibular and visual systems
   (b) Efferents direct to motor centres in brain stem and spinal cord

2. Cerebellar hemispheres
   (a) Afferents from cortical sensorimotor association areas
   (b) Efferents to thalamic (VA) motor centres and thence to motor cortex

3. Cerebellum in general
   (a) All **afferents** reach the cerebellar cortex by dual pathways (**mossy** and **climbing fibre systems**, of undetermined functional significance)
   (b) Single **efferent** pathway from cerebellar cortex via **axons of Purkinje cells** which act by exclusive inhibitory synapses (by GABA transmission) on the neurons of the cerebellar nuclei (modulation of motor activity by up- or down-regulation of inhibition).

Actions of parts of the cerebellum on motor functions

	Functions
Vermis	Control and correction of components of postural supporting mechanisms and movements (posture, tone, equilibration)
Pars intermedia	Directional control of slower aimed movements and coordination with supportive postural measures
Hemispheres of cerebellum	Performance of rapid directed movements initiated by cerebral hemispheres; cooperation in the learning and performance of rapid directed motor actions devoid of feed-back (ballistic movements), e.g. articulation, eye movement saccades, performance of music, sport

NEUROLOGICAL SYMPTOMS AND SYNDROMES

Disorders of cerebellar function

1. Neocerebellum (cerebellar hemispheres)
   Ipsilateral ataxia of limbs (upper > lower), hypotonia and hyporeflexia, dysmetria, dysdiadochokinesia, increasing intention tremor (2–3/s) on approaching target, rebound phenomenon, visual fixation dysmetria, dysarthria (paravermal segment of left hemisphere).

2. Vestibulocerebellum (archicerebellum, flocculonodular lobe)
   Stance and gait ataxia, trunk and head ataxia (also in sitting position), liability to fall over, saccadic eye pursuit movements, abnormal vestibuloocular reflex, rebound and downbeat nystagmus (increasing on lateral gaze), dysarthria.

3. Spinocerebellum (palaeocerebellum, anterior lobe of hemispheres and upper vermis)
   Uncertainty of stance and gait, with forward and backward swaying, patient does not quite fall, marked ataxia in heel–knee–shin test, 3 Hz body tremor, saccadic pursuit eye movements.

Important causes

- Tumour, infarction, haemorrhage
- System degenerations
- Alcoholic and nutritional cerebellar degeneration.

MEMORIX NEUROLOGY

Cerebellum viewed from above

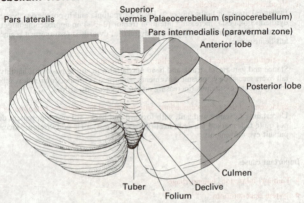

Cerebellum viewed from below

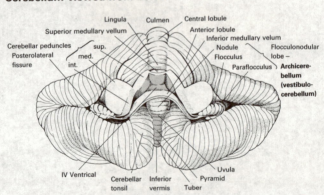

NEUROLOGICAL SYMPTOMS AND SYNDROMES

Schema of autonomic nervous system
Origin, distribution and areas of innervation
(Reproduced after Jänig, W. *Vegetatives Nevensystem*, in: *Grundriss der Neurophysiologie*, 6th edn, (ed. Schmidt, R.F.), published by Springer, Berlin, 1987.)

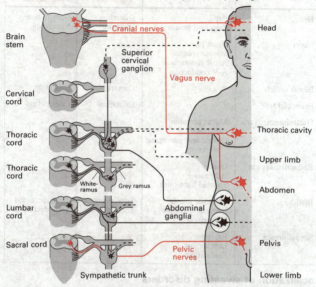

	Description/commentary
Sympathetic	Preganglionic neurons in thoracic and upper lumbar spinal cord (black); preganglionic axons (B and C fibres) terminate in the paravertebral ganglia of the sympathetic trunk or in unpaired abdominal ganglia; the long postganglionic axons (C fibres) go to effector organs
Parasympathetic	Preganglionic neurons are in brain stem and sacral cord (red); the preganglionic axons (B and C fibres) end in parasympathetic ganglia near the effector organs which are reached by short postganglionic axons (C fs.)
Intestinal plexuses	Myenteric (Auerbach's) plexus and submucous (Meissner's) plexus: both contain sensory, motor and interneurons; main function is control of gastrointestinal tract; it is modulated by sympathetic and parasympathetic inflow

Functions of sympathetic and parasympathetic nervous systems

		Sympathetic	Parasympathetic
Eye	Pupil	Dilatation	Constriction
	Palpebral fissure	Widening	Narrowing
Heart	Heart rate	↑	↓
	Minute volume	↑	↓
	Atrial contraction	↑	↓
	A-V conduction	↑	↓
Blood vessels		Constriction	Dilatation
Bronchial tree		Dilatation	Constriction
Gastrointestinal tract	Mucus secretion	↓	↑
	Peristalsis	↓	↑
	Gastric and pancreatic secretion	↓	↑
Endocrine system	Insulin	↑	↓
	Adrenaline	↑	↓
	Thyroid hormones	↑	↓
Bladder	Detrusor muscle	Tone decreased	Tone increased
	Internal sphincter	Tone increased	Tone decreased
	Micturition	↓	↑
Sexual organs	Erection	↓	↑
	Lubrication	↓	↑
	Ejaculation	↑	↓

Localization of sweating disorders

- Hemianhidrosis: Lesion of central sympathetic connections (preservation of Pilocarpine sweat response)
- Anhidrosis of half of face: Lesion of cervical sympathetic
- Anhidrosis of lower half of body: Spinal cord lesion between T3 and L2
- Anhidrosis of upper quadrant excluding face: Sympathetic chain level T4–T5
- Anhidrosis of upper quadrant plus Horner's syndrome: sympathetic chain including stellate ganglion
- Anhidrosis of upper quadrant without Horner's syndrome: sympathetic chain below stellate ganglion (T3)
- Horner's syndrome with preservation of sweating: C8–T2 lesion proximal to sympathetic chain
- Anhidrosis of lower quadrant (hind quarter): Sympathetic chain lesion at level T12
- Anhidrosis below knee: Sympathetic chain lesion at level L2.

NB Root lesions C5 to T2 do not cause disorders of sweating. Disorders of thermoregulation plus loss of pharmacological sweating suggest plexus or peripheral nerve lesions.

NEUROLOGICAL SYMPTOMS AND SYNDROMES

Functions of sympathetic nerves and localization of sweating disorders

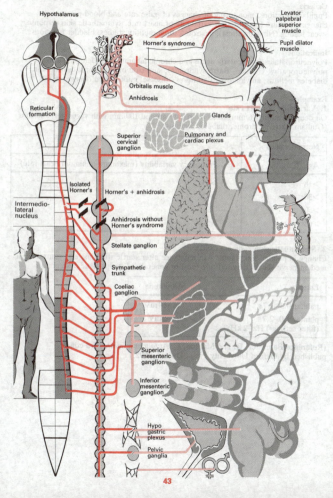

Autonomic function assessment

Criteria
Pupillary reactions, monitoring of changes of pulse rate and blood pressure on changing posture (orthostasis), variability of heart rate, sympathetic skin response, sweat testing (Ninhydrin test), gastrointestinal motility studies, bladder functions.

Indications
Polyneuropathies (particularly acute and chronic inflammatory demyelinating polyneuropathy, Guillain–Barré syndrome), suspicion of autonomic disorders in diabetes mellitus, amyloidosis, Parkinson's disease, multisystem degenerations.

Examples
1. Variability of heart rate
On deep breathing (6/min) fixed heart rate around 100/min with vagus nerve lesions (Guillain Barré syndrome, diabetes mellitus).

Normal values	
Age	Frequency variability (maximum-minimum heart rate)
>18	>15
>30	>11
>50	>9
>65	>5

2. Sympathetic skin response (SSR)
Change in palmar and plantar skin resistance after startle stimulus, e.g. contralateral median nerve shock; may indicate focal or generalized sympathetic dysfunction.

Latency	Amplitude
palmar 0.3–1.7 s	0.4–10 mV
plantar 1.0–2.7 s (filter setting 1 Hz–2 kHz)	0.2–5 mV

(Reference Bannister, R. and Mathias, C. *Autonomic failure*, 3rd edn, published by Oxford University Press, Oxford, 1992.)

Tests of sweating

Ninhydrin test
(Moberg, E. (1958) Objective methods for determining the functional value of sensibility in the hand. *Journal of Bone and Joint Surgery*, **40B**, 454–76.)

1. Clean and dry area of skin to be tested.
2. Press skin against sheet of white paper and draw outline of finger without impinging examiner's fingerprints (gloves).
3. Moisten paper with 1% solution of Ninhydrin in acetone, adding a few drops of glacial acetic acid just prior to test.
4. Dry the paper in oven (100°C).
5. Fix in solution of methanol 95%, distilled water 5%, copper nitrate 1% plus drops of concentrated nitric acid.

Chinizarin (starch) test
(Guttmann, L. (1940) Disturbances of sweat secretion. *Journal of Neurology, Neurosurgery and Psychiatry*, **3**, 197–210.)

Prepare dry powder mixture of Chinizarin (quinizarin) sodium 35 g, Sodium Carbonate 30 g, rice starch 30 g. Dust the reddish-grey powder over skin to be tested and place under heat cradle for 15–45 min.

For provocation of **thermoregulatory sweating** apply radiant heat, or use sauna, but beware risk of heat injury to anaesthetized skin.

For provocation of **pharmacological sweating** inject Pilocarpine 10 mg subcutaneously and allow 15 min for effect.

MEMORIX NEUROLOGY

Bladder function
Bladder and retaining musculature

	Fibre type	Innervation	Nerve	Effect
Detrusor muscle	Smooth	Parasympathetic (S3, S4)	Pelvic nerves	Bladder contraction
		Sympathetic (T11–L2)	Hypogastric nerve	Relaxation of bladder muscle
Internal sphincter	Smooth	Sympathetic	Hypogastric nerve	Narrowing bladder neck
External sphincter	Striated	Somatic (S2–S4)	Pudendal nerve	Voluntary interruption of flow of urine
Pelvic floor muscles	Striated	Somatic and parasympathetic	Pudendal and pelvic nerves	Continence maintenance during filling

Micturition centres
Pontine micturition centre: reticular formation
Sacral micturition centre: conus medullaris (S2–S4)

Bladder disorders
(From Möbius, E. (1993) Neurologische Aspekte von Blasenfunctionsstörungen. Jahrbuch Neurologie Biermann Zülpich)

1. **Detrusor hyperreflexia** (cerebral bladder disinhibition) with superior frontal gyrus lesions, or subcortical lesions (basal ganglia, hypothalamus)
   Clinically: urgency, frequency, urge incontinence, no residual urine
   Treatment: oxybutynine, imipramine, desipramine;
   if ineffective: urinal, incontinence pants/pads, possibly in-dwelling catheter.

2. **Detrusor-sphincter dyssynergia** (spastic bladder) with supranuclear cord lesions (above level of conus medullaris).
   Clinically: 'staccato' micturition, little or moderate amount residual urine frequency with urge- or reflex-incontinence, occasionally retention
   Treatment: bladder training (suprapubic pressure, perianal tactile stimulation); residual urine >100 ml and/or recurrent infections of urinary tract: intermittent (self-)catheterization and drug inhibition of detrusor (oxybutynin, imipramine, desipramine).

3. **Detrusor areflexia** (flaccid bladder) with lesion of sacral micturition centre, or of peripheral bladder innervation, or during stage of spinal shock
   Clinically: poor voluntary emptying, retention, high residual, overflow incontinence, possibly neurogenic stress incontinence
   Treatment: intermittent (self-)catheterization or transient suprapubic drainage; attempts at passive emptying by abdominal pressure and Crédé manoeuvre.

NEUROLOGICAL SYMPTOMS AND SYNDROMES

Neurogenic bladder disorders
Schema of investigation and management

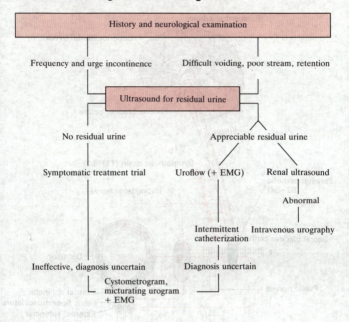

MEMORIX NEUROLOGY

Neuroanatomy of bladder disorders

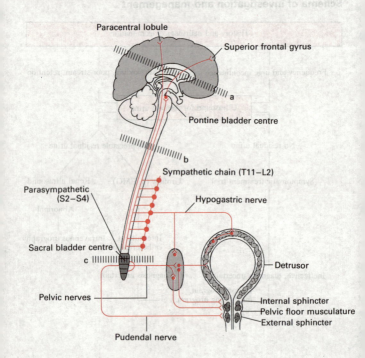

NEUROLOGICAL SYMPTOMS AND SYNDROMES

Neurogenic bladder disorders: causes and treatment

Site of lesion	Type of bladder disorder	Causes	Treatment
(a) Suprapontine	Central disinhibition of bladder reflexes (detrusor hyper-reflexia, uncontrollable urge and urge incontinence)	Dementing illnesses, trauma, ischaemia, multiple sclerosis, hydrocephalus	Oxybutynin, imipramine, desipramine; if persistent incontinence urethral, in-dwelling catheter
(b) Spinal cord (suprasacral)	Spinal shock: detrusor areflexia with overflow incontinence Later, or incomplete lesions: spastic bladder with detrusor-sphincter dyssynergia; urge or reflex incontinence	Trauma, transverse myelitis, ischaemia Multiple sclerosis, tumour, spinal degenerations AV malformations	Intermittent catheterization or suprapubic drainage Training (suprapubic pressure, perianal stimulation; if incontinent, >100 ml residual or recurrent infections: intermittent catheterization (+ anticholinergics)
(c) Conus, cauda and peripheral nerves	Detrusor areflexia with acute or chronic retention, overflow incontinence, neurogenic stress incontinence	Trauma, central lumbar disc prolapse, tumour, polyneuropathy, malformations, tabes, postoperative pelvic plexus lesions, sacral radiculopathy	Intermittent (self)catheterization, possibly suprapubic drainage Passive emptying by abdominal compression (Crédé's manoeuvre)

Lesion sites (a), (b) and (c) shown in diagram on p. 48

Cortex: integrative functions
Integrative functions of the central nervous system

1. **Circadian periodicity** of sleep – waking cycle
2. **Consciousness**
3. **Speech**
4. **Thought** (understanding, reason)
5. **Memory** including learning and recollection
6. **Motivation**
7. **Emotion**

The limbic system takes a decisive role in functions 6 and 7, the neocortex in functions 1–5. Certain cortical areas have special tasks that are often in only one hemisphere (hemisphere specialization), e.g. motor and sensory speech centres (Broca's and Wernicke's)

Lateral view of left hemisphere cortex (frontal, temporal, parietal and occipital cortex)
(Reproduced after Schmidt, R.F. Integrative Leistungen des CNS, in *Physiologie des Menschen*, 24th edn, (eds, Schmidt, R.F. and Thews, G., Springer, Berlin, 1990.)

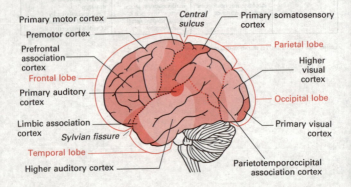

Integrative functions of the three cortical association areas of humans

Association cortex	Integrative function
Parietotemporoccipital	Sensory speech functions, higher sensory tasks, e.g. matching auditory and visual information
Prefrontal	Higher motor tasks, e.g. movement strategies, acquired control of inborn behaviour patterns
Limbic	Motivation, emotional–affective aspects of behaviour

NEUROLOGICAL SYMPTOMS AND SYNDROMES

Grades of anosognosia

Anosognosia = failure to recognize neurological deficit.
Grade 1: unaware of defect, feels normal,
Grade 2: unaware of defect but aware of consequences, e.g. of bumping into things,
Grade 3: aware of changed environment,
Grade 4: aware of disordered function but not of its cause,
Grade 5: aware of disordered function but misinterprets cause,
Grade 6: full insight into disordered function.

Neglect: neglect of part of anatomy or of external space.
Disconnection: interruption.

Important neuropsychological disorders

1. **Alexia:** disorder of reading through faulty recognition of letters (literal alexia), or of words (verbal alexia). Lesion site: left angular gyrus; in alexia without agraphia: left visual cortex and posterior corpus callosum (posterior disconnection syndrome).
2. **Agraphia:** disorder of writing through faulty construction of letters (constructional agraphia), or faulty choice or order of letters, syllables, or words; often an epiphenomenon of aphasia. Demonstration by writing test. Lesion site: left angular gyrus.
3. **Acalculia:** disorder of ability to calculate. Lesion site: left angular gyrus.
4. **Amnesia:** disorder of storage of memories (recording defect), and/or of recall of memories (defect of old memories). Separate testing for ability to record and for old memories. Lesion site: medial temporal lobe or paramedian thalamus.
5. **Anosognosia:** failure of awareness of neurological deficit, e.g. of hemiparesis or of cortical blindness. Lesion site: right parietotemporal.
6. **Aphasia:** disorder of central speech mechanism. For accurate classification assess spontaneous speech, naming and repetition of heard speech (cf. table on p. 52).
7. **Ideomotor apraxia:** disorder of sequence of willed movements by lapses, perseveration, distortion (parapraxia). Demonstration by tests of willed complex movements. Lesion site: left parietal lobe or left premotor cortex; when only left half of body affected: anterior corpus callosum (anterior disconnection syndrome).
8. **Constructional apraxia:** disorder of design in space of constructional movements, e.g. in handicrafts, building, drawing. Demonstrate by copying of drawings. The overall arrangement of the drawing is disjointed, and/or details are wrongly placed. Lesion site: left or right parietal lobe.
9. **Neglect syndrome:** stimuli of varying modalities are disregarded which originate from one side of body, or from one side of external space (usually left side). Demonstrate by bisection of a line (midpoint shifted to right), or by copying (when details of e.g. left half are left out). Lesion site: parietal lobe, rarely frontal lobe contralateral to affected side.
10. **Object agnosia:** failure of recognition of objects specifically by one sensory modality (usually visual) which cannot be explained by a disorder of perception such as a visual field defect. Demonstrate by naming test (faulty naming through failure of recognition). Lesion site: posterior temporal lobe, usually bilateral.
11. **Disorientation in space:** disordered perception of localization of objects in space, or of the spatial relationship of objects to each other. Demonstrate by orientation test using clock face devoid of digits. Lesion site: right parietal lobe.

MEMORIX NEUROLOGY

Speech: Aphasia

Aphasia	Spontaneous speech	Understanding of speech	Naming	Repeating speech	Other	Localization
Broca	Telegrammatic WF/AG	Minor disorder	SP/WF	PP	(NL)	3rd frontal convolution
Wernicke	fluent/PG	Severe disorder	SP	(PP)	Logorrhoea (NL)	1st temporal convolution
Amnesic	WF	Normal	WF (SP)	Normal	–	Non-specific
Global	AG/NL/Aut	Severe disorder	Impossible (SP)	Impossible (PP)	–	Anterior and posterior middle cerebral artery territory
Conductive	fluent	Minor disorder	Normal	Impossible (PP)	–	Subcortical middle cerebral artery territory
Transcortical motor	poor	Normal	Normal	(PP)	–	Premotor cortex
Transcortical sensory	fluent	Severe disorder	SP	Normal	Echolalia	Occipitotemporal

Abbreviations:
AG: agrammatism, 'basic' syntax, 'pidgin', lack of quantities, qualifications etc.
Aut: automatism, constantly recurring utterances
NL: neologisms
PG: paragrammatism, complex syntax with wrong quantities, qualifications etc.
PP: phonemic paraphasia, distortion of words by wrong sounds (phonemes)
SP: semantic paraphasia, choice of word with meaning deviant from intended word
WF: word finding difficulty, hesitant flow from frequent search for words

Cortical areas involved in speech based on Geschwind's model from brain lesions (subcortical connections not shown in illustration)
(Reproduced after Kolb, B. and Winshaw, I.Q. *Fundamentals of human neuropsychology*; Published by Freeman, New York, 1985.)

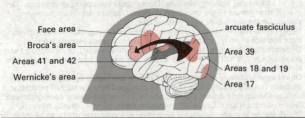

1. Spoken word → areas 41, 42 → Wernicke's (area 22) → hearing and understanding word.
2. Understanding → Wernicke's → Broca's → face → cranial nerves → speaking.
3. Written word → area 17 → area 18, 19 → area 39 (angular gyrus) → Wernicke's → reading.

Higher mental function testing
Bedside neuropsychological testing

Language testing
- Repetition of words and sentences
- Naming of common objects
- Reading of letters, words, sentences
- Writing of name, address, to dictation
- Spontaneous speech

Visuospatial
- Recognition of objects
- Copying simple geometric figures
- Time on clock face
- Halving of lines

Praxis
- Miming of movements and copying
- Movements on verbal instruction ('touch left ear with right thumb')

Memory
- Repetition of simple numbers (at least six digits)
- Repetition of sentences (e.g. Babcock's 'What makes a country powerful and strong is a good and plentiful supply of wood'); short-term memory: past personal; long-term memory: world events

Mental arithmetic
- Simple additions and subtractions
- Subtract 7 from 100 (serially)

NB   All tests must allow for initial intelligence and educational level, and for any disorder of language (dysphasia).

Minimental test scoring (in absence of dysphasia)

	Score
Reproduced from Folstein, M.F., Folstein, S.E. and McHugh, P.R. (1975) Minimental State. *Journal of Psychiatric Research*, **12**, 189.	
Orientation (time, date, day of week, month, year)	5
Name of ward, of hospital, district, town, country	5
Registration: name 3 common objects and repeat (see below)	3
Attention/calculation: 100 − 7, and continue × 5 to 65	5
Recall three objects named above	3
Language: name 2 common objects, e.g. pencil, watch	2
Repetition of 'no ifs, no ands, no buts'	1
Three-stage command: 'take paper, fold it in half and put on table'	3
Written command 'shut your eyes'	1
Write a sentence: if result meaningful with verb and subject	1
Visuospatial: copy drawing of 2 intersecting pentagons	1
Maximal score	30

Score: <20 probably demented; 21–25 equivocal; >25 probably normal

Cognitive differences of the two hemispheres

Differential cognitive strategies of the cerebral hemispheres in right-handed persons
(Reproduced after Schmidt, R.F. Integrative Leistungen des CNS, in *Physiologie des Menschen*, 24th edn, (eds Schmidt, R.F. and Thews, G.), Springer, Heidelberg, 1990.)

Left	Right
Verbal	Spatial, physiognomic
Analytic	Holistic, global, 'Gestalt', Sythetic, 'musical'
Sequential	Simultaneous, parallel
Focused	Diffuse
Finding similarities	Finding differences
Abstract, conceptual	Concrete, corporeal
Rational	Intuitive
'conscious'	'unconscious'
Declarative recollection	Reflective recollection
Stronger reaction to positive emotional stimuli	Stronger reaction to negative emotional stimuli
Lesion: depressivity	Lesion: equanimity, euphoria
Epileptic focus 'forced laughter' 'gelastic epilepsy'	Epileptic focus 'forced crying' (?) 'dacrystic epilepsy'
Perception of 'myself in the world'	Perception of 'the world in myself'

NEUROLOGICAL SYMPTOMS AND SYNDROMES

Dysarthrias
Dysarthrias from neurological causes

(Reproduced from Berlit, P. (1987) Dysarthrien bei neurolog. Erkrankungen; published in *Nervenarzt*, **58**, 272–8.)

Classification by clinical features

Peripheral dysarthria (flaccid)	
Diffuse	Polyneuritis, myopathy, myasthenia gravis
Focal	Isolated cranial nerve lesions
Central dysarthria	
Spastic	Pseudobulbar palsy
Ataxic	Cerebellar lesion
Bradykinetic	Parkinsonism
Hyperkinetic	Chorea, dystonia
Complex forms	
Spastic–flaccid	Motor neuron disease
Spastic–ataxic–bradykinetic	Wilson's disease
Various combinations	Disseminated encephalomyelitis

Classification of dysarthrias by site of lesion

	Common clinical causes
Hemispheric (cortical) dysarthria:	
Lesion of lower precentral gyrus	Infarction, tumour
Variant: frontal dysarthria	General paralysis of the insane, trauma
Corticobulbar dysarthria	Pseudobulbar palsy
Extrapyramidal dysarthria	
Basal ganglia lesions	Parkinsonism, chorea, dystonia
Cerebellar dysarthria	
Cerebellar lesions (left paravermal)	Disseminated encephalomyelitis, infarction, tumour, multiple sclerosis, hereditary and acquired cerebellar degenerations
Cranial nerve dysarthria	
Nuclear lesions	Motor neuron disease, tumours, poliomyelitis, infarction, syringobulbia
Peripheral lesions	Polyneuritis cranialis, tumour of skull-base (Garcin's syndrome), trauma, tuberculosis
Muscular dysarthria	
Neuromuscular junction	Myasthenia gravis
Muscle diseases	Muscular dystrophies, myositis, dystrophia myotonica

Central and neuromuscular disorders of respiration

(Reproduced after Mummenthaler, M. (1991) Neurologische Atemstörungen. *Extracta Psychiatrica*, **5**, 21.)

Central disorders of respiration

Type of breathing	Occurs in	Site of lesion/mechanism
Cheyne–Stokes (periodic) respiration	Hypoxia during sleep, poisoning, cerebral ischaemia, haemorrhage, encephalitis	Diencephalon, diffuse deepseated hemisphere lesions
Biot's (intermittent, ataxic) respiration	Brain trauma, raised intracranial pressure, posterior fossa lesions	Dorsomedial medulla
Kussmaul respiration ('air hunger')	Diabetic coma	Non-respiratory (metabolic) acidosis
Apnoea (respiratory arrest in inspiration)	Cerebral (vertebro-basilar) ischaemia, posterior fossa lesions	Central/caudal pons and dorsal tegmentum
Ondine's curse (temporary loss of automatic breathing during sleep)	Acute disorders of medulla oblongata	Reticulospinal projections of medulla oblongata
Central hyperventilation	Craniocerebral trauma	Rostral brain stem, rostral tegmentum, reticular formation
Gasping	Craniocerebral trauma, prematurity, raised intracranial pressure (coning)	Reticular formation

Designation		Occurs in
Normal respiration At rest		
Cheyne–Stokes (periodic) respiration		Hypoxia during sleep, poisoning
Biot's respiration		Cerebral trauma, raised intracranial pressure
Kussmaul respiration (air hunger)		Non-respiratory (metabolic) acidosis
Gasping		Prematurity, brain damage

NEUROLOGICAL SYMPTOMS AND SYNDROMES

Neuromuscular disorders

Type of disorder	Diseases	Special features
1. Anterior horn cell disorders	Acute anterior poliomyelitis	Acute respiratory failure, later possible chronic failure from hypoventilation or scoliosis
	Chronic spinal muscular atrophies	
	Infantile (Werdnig Hoffmann disease)	Increasing respiratory failure during first two years of life
	Intermediary form	Juvenile or adult respiratory insufficiency
	Chronic proximal spinal muscular atrophy (Kugelberg–Welander)	No respiratory insufficiency
	Motor neuron disease	Progressive respiratory failure in adults
2. Anterior spinal roots	Acute polyradiculopathy (Guillain–Barré)	May produce acute (reversible) respiratory failure
3. (Bilateral) C4 lesion	Bilateral diaphragmatic palsy	Respiratory insufficiency on minimal exertion
4. Peripheral nerves	Bilateral phrenic palsy	e.g. with mediastinal tumours, diaphragmatic palsy with exertional respiratory insufficiency
	Polyneuropathies	Hardly ever cause respiratory insufficiency
5. Motor end-plate disorders	Myasthenia gravis	May cause severe respiratory insufficiency
	Drugs, toxins	e.g. curare and other muscle relaxants used in anaesthesia, neurotoxic agents
6. Muscle disorders	Progressive muscular dystrophies	Chronic respiratory insufficiency only in Duchenne and Becker forms
	Hypokalaemia	Very rarely mild respiratory insufficiency
	Polymyositis	Very rarely mild respiratory insufficiency

Causes of disorders of consciousness

(Reproduced from Berlit, P. *Neurologie in der Praxis*; published by V.C.H., Weinheim, 1988.)

		Slowly progressive disorder of consciousness	Sudden loss of consciousness	Increasing confusion
Intracranial	Trauma	Subdural haematoma	Extradural haematoma, contusion	Oedema, subdural haematoma, post-traumatic confusional state
	Tumour	Oedema	Fit, coning, haemorrhage, obstructive hydrocephalus	Oedema
	Vascular	Infarction with mass effect, intracerebral bleed	Brain stem infarction, major intracerebral bleed, subarachnoid bleed	Postinfarct or postbleed oedema Transient global amnesia
	Inflammation	Bacterial meningitis Encephalitis	Raised intracranial pressure from brain abscess Oedema and bleeding with meningo-encephalitis	Encephalitis
	Toxic	Wernicke's disease Central pontine myelinolysis	Central pontine myelinolysis Corpus callosum lesion	Alcoholism, Wernicke–Korsakov state Other drugs
	Epilepsy		Grand mal, complex partial seizures	Psychomotor attacks, petit mal status
Extracranial	Metabolic	Electrolyte disorders (Na, K) Hypoxia, acidosis/alkalosis, renal and hepatic failure	Electrolyte disorders (Ca, Na) Porphyria	Hypoxia, electrolyte disorders, dehydration, Hypo- and hyperthermia, porphyria
	Hormonal	Hyperglycaemia Hypothyroidism Hypopituitarism	Hypoglycaemia	Hyperglycaemia Hyperthyroidism
	CV and respiratory systems	Blood loss Anaemia Hypoventilation	Fall in blood pressure Cardiac dysrrhythmia Carotid sinus syndrome, pulmonary embolism	Anaemia
	Psychiatric	Catatonia	Psychogenic fainting	Dementias
	Toxic	Sedatives, psychotropic, neuroleptic, anticonvulsant drugs, carbon monoxide, heavy metals	Sedatives, hypnotics, carbon monoxide, drugs	Heavy metals, drugs

NEUROLOGICAL SYMPTOMS AND SYNDROMES

Mental state assessment

(Reference: Hodges, J.R. *Cognitive assessment for clinicians*; published by Oxford University Press, Oxford, 1994.)

1. **Conscious level:** retardation, somnolence, delirium, twilight state.

2. **Orientation:** time, place, person.

3. **Powers of perception and concentration:** concrete and abstract notions, interpretation.

4. **Ability to record, short- and long-term memory:** memory gaps (possibly confabulation), perseveration, recollection of numbers and personal data.

5. **Progression of ideas – formal thinking:** inhibited, circumstantial, retarded, perseverating, incoherent, twisted, accelerated (flight of ideas), halting of ideas, constriction, autism, judgmental ability, decisiveness, exaggerated ideas.

6. **Basic mood and affective reactivity:** lability of affect, emotional incontinence, inner disquiet, tension, irritability, querulousness, euphoria, anxiety, sadness (depression), hopelessness, lack of affect, antagonism, loss of self-regard, notions of guilt and poverty, doubts of survival

7. **Psychotic symptoms:** hallucinations, manic ideas, personality disorders, suicidal ideas, compulsions, phobias

8. **Simulation, exaggeration**

9. **Assessment criteria of psychic disorders with an organic basis**
   (Reproduced after Hierholzer, K. and Schmidt, R. *Pathophysiologie des Menschen*; published by V.C.H., Weinheim, 1991.)

Range of psychic functions and their disorders

Consciousness	Somnolence → stupor → coma

Alertness	Distractability, perseveration
	  Circumstantiality, discursiveness
	  Incoherence

Perception/recognition	Illusions, hallucinations, agnosia
Interest/motivation	Apathy, impulsiveness

Memory	Amnesia (occasionally with confabulation), disorientation for time → situation → place → own personality
	Stages of processing: Engram formation (learning)
	    Recording (retention)
	    Reproduction (recall)
	Qualities: Declaratory (a) semantic: facts
	                        (b) episodic: events
	    Reflective: strategies
	Duration Short-term
	    Long-term

Intelligence	Dementia
	  Verbal
	  Non-verbal

Affect	Lability of affect, depression, euphoria, irritability

Mental disorders with an organic basis

(Modified from Huber, G. *Psychiatrie*, 4th edn, published by Schattauer, Stuttgart, 1987.)

Acute mental disorders

	Main symptoms	Examples
Episodic syndromes	Reduced spontaneity; disordered affect (depressive, manic), pseudoneurasthenic, hysteria-like Productive: expansive–confabulatory, paranoid–hallucinatory, catatonic Hallucinations: auditory, visual, tactile Amnestic: acute Korsakov state 'Orientated twilight state'	Intoxications Metabolic disorders Inflammation (encephalitis, parainfectious) Brain trauma Vascular Epilepsy (ictal or postictal)
Impaired consciousness	Graded: slowing, somnolence, stupor, coma Qualitative–productive: confusion, delirium, twilight state	Trauma, metabolic disorders, encephalitis, space occupying lesions Intoxications, cerebral ischaemia, epilepsy

Chronic mental disorders

Chronic pseudoneur-asthenic syndrome (failing intellect)	Altered affective responses (increased irritability) and vulnerability (poor concentration, fatiguability)	Post-traumatic Postischaemic Postencephalitic
Organic personality change	Accentuation or diminution of character traits Alteration of basic mood or drive Retardation Types: apathetic, torpid euphoric, fussy irritable, irascible, disinhibited chronic paranoid hallucinatory syndrome	Chronic epilepsy Cerebral tumour Postencephalitic Degenerations and multisystem atrophies
Dementia	Memory disorders (recollection, recording new data) Intellectual decline (critical, comprehensive, logical, formation and combination of ideas) Specific variant: chronic Korsakov state	Alzheimer's disease, senile (Alzheimer-type) dementia, multi-infarct dementia, general paralysis of the insane, chronic alcoholism

NEUROLOGICAL SYMPTOMS AND SYNDROMES

Brain syndromes

- Angular gyrus syndrome (Gerstmann syndrome): finger agnosia, acalculia, right-left disorientation, agraphia and alexia (tumour, infarction, trauma)
- Athetosis: sluggish writhing hyperkinesia of distal parts of limbs, variable muscle tone (infarction, haemorrhage, anoxia)
- Balint's syndrome (mind blindness): disordered visual perception from damage to association fibres between cortical visual centres (tumour, infarction)
- Ballismus: see Hemiballismus
- Bulbar syndrome: coma, dilated and unreactive pupils, apnoea, circulatory anomalies, muscles flaccid (trauma, tumour, infarction)
- Cerebellar hemisphere syndrome: ipsilateral limb ataxia, dysdiadochokinesis, hypotonia, gaze nystagmus (tumour, infarction, haemorrhage)
- Cerebellar vermis syndrome: trunk and gait ataxia, muscle hypotonia, saccadic gaze pursuit, dysarthria (tumour, atrophies)
- Cerebellopontine angle syndrome: deafness, tinnitus (with acoustic neuroma), VII and V nerve deficits, ipsilateral cerebellar and contralateral pyramidal signs (meningioma, dermoid)
- Choreic syndromes: involuntary rapid random jerks of facial and of groups of limb muscles (cessation during sleep), hypotonicity of muscles, persistent knee extension on tapping knee jerk (ischaemia, inflammation, degenerative, toxic)
- Clivus syndrome: ipsilateral oculomotor pressure palsy (including pupil) (tumour, haemorrhage)
- Corpus callosum syndromes: (a) Rostral: apraxic left hand, contralateral grasp reflex (b) Central: dysgraphia left hand (c) Splenium: alexia, homonymous hemianopia (glioma, corpus callosum degeneration)
- Decerebrate syndrome: coma, synergism of flexor and extensor muscles, autonomic disorders, oculomotor and pupillary unreactivity (trauma, tumour)
- Disconnection syndromes: neuropsychological disorders (often agnosic) from lesions of interhemispheric association tracts. e.g. lesion of splenium plus left occipital lobe (left posterior cerebral infarct): right homonymous hemianopia, alexia and achromatopsia; or, lesion of association tracts from left to right motor cortex and left arcuate fasciculus: right-sided ideomotor apraxia with sympathetic left hand dyspraxia (Liepmann)
- Dystonic syndrome: variable hypertonicity and contraction of muscle groups lasting seconds, rotatory movements of neck and trunk (ischaemia, toxic, degenerative)
- Foramen jugulare syndrome (Siebenmann syndrome): Lesion of cranial nerves IX, X, XI (tumour, trauma, jugular vein thrombosis)
- Foramen magnum syndrome: episodic head and neck pain, vomiting. autonomic disorders, abnormal head postures, ocular bobbing, bulbar dysarthria (tumour, craniocervical anomalies)
- Frontal lobe syndrome: personality change, altered drive, lack of judgment, fits (focal motor, adversive), contralateral paresis, motor aphasia dominant hemisphere) (trauma, tumour, infarction)
- Hemiballismus: involuntary hurling hyperkinesis due to interruption of tracts from subthalamic nucleus (corpus Luysii) to globus pallidus (infarction, haemorrhage)

- Hertwig-Magendie syndrome (skew deviation): down-and-in squint of one eye, or up-and-out by other eye, from damaged trochlear decussation (tumour, haemorrhage)
- Hypothalamic syndrome: diabetes insipidus, sleep and autonomic (e.g. temperature) disorders.
- Insular cortex syndrome: focal epilepsy, abnormal trunk sensations (tumour)
- Internuclear ophthalmoplegia: see p. 9
- Klüver-Bucy syndrome: oral tendencies (mouthing of objects), reduced drive, amnesia, occ. sexual disinhibition (bi-temporal medial temporal lobe damage from infarcts, trauma, atrophies, e.g. Pick's disease)
- Medullary syndromes
Lateral infarctions
  1. Avellis syndrome: ipsilateral IX and X with contralateral sensory-motor hemiparesis
  2. Cestan–Chenais syndrome: ipsilateral Horner's and hemiataxia with paresis of IX and X and contralateral sensory-motor hemiparesis
  3. Schmidt syndrome: ipsilateral paresis of IX, X, XI and XII with contralateral sensory-motor hemiparesis
  4. Tapia syndrome: ipsilateral paresis of IX, X and XII with contralateral sensory-motor hemiparesis
  5. Vernet syndrome: ipsilateral paresis of IX, X and XI with contralateral sensory-motor hemiparesis

  Posterolateral medullary infarction (Wallenberg's syndrome): ipsilateral Horner's, hemiataxia, nystagmus, trigeminal sensory loss, paresis of IX and X, with contralateral dissociated sensory loss below (posterior cerebellar or vertebral artery ischaemia)

  Inferior medullary infarction (Jackson's syndrome): ipsilateral hypoglossal paresis with contralateral motor hemiparesis
- Mills' palsy: slowly progressive and entirely motor, contralateral hemiparesis from localized precentral cortical atrophy
- Midbrain syndrome: coma, autonomic and respirstory disorders, extensor spasticity, oculomotor palsies (trauma, tumour, infarction)
- Nothnagel syndrome: ipsilateral oculomotor palsy with contralateral hemiataxia (midbrain tectus infarction or tumour); see Parinaud's syndrome
- Occipital lobe syndrome: contralateral homonymous hemianopia, visual hallucinations, dyslexia, visual agnosia (tumour, infarct, haemorrhage, trauma)
- Olfactory groove syndrome: unilateral or bilateral anosmia, personality change (tumour)
- Orbital apex syndrome: lesions of II, III, IV and VI and V^1 (trauma, tumour)
- Parasagittal syndrome: contralateral or bilateral lower limb palsy with micturition disorders (tumour)
- Parietal lobe syndrome: contralateral sensory disturbance, homonymous hemianopia, inattention, focal sensory seizures, spatial disorientation (non-dominant hemisphere), amnestic aphasia (dominant hemisphere) (tumour, infarction, haemorrhage)
- Parinaud's syndrome: upward gaze palsy, poor convergence, pupils abnormal (dorsal midbrain tumour or infarction); see Nothnagel syndrome
- Parkinson's syndrome: hypokinesia, rigidity, tremor
- Persistent vegetative state

MEMORIX NEUROLOGY

Brain syndromes (continued)

- Petrous apex (Gradenigo's syndrome): VI palsy, reduced sensation V^1, deafness (tumour, petrous bone infection)

- Red nucleus syndromes
  Upper rubral syndrome of Chiray–Foix–Nicolesco: contralateral hemihyperkinesia (midbrain-rubral infarction)
  Upper rubral syndrome of Benedikt: oculomotor palsy and contralateral hemiataxia (midbrain-rubral infarction)
  Lower rubral syndrome of Claude: oculomotor palsy with contralateral hemiataxia (midbrain-rubral infarction)

- Retropharyngeal syndrome of Villaret: lesion of IX, X, XI and XII plus Horner's syndrome (tumours)

- Skull base (Garcin's) syndrome: unilateral paresis of nerves V–XII (tumours, inflammations of skull base)

- Tectal syndromes (infarcts of tectum pontis):
  Rostral tectal (Raymond–Céstan) syndrome: horizontal gaze palsy towards side of lesion, contralateral sensory disorder
  Caudal tectal (Gasperini) syndrome: ipsilateral paresis of V, VI, VII and VIII and contralateral sensory disorder
  Caudal tectal (Millard–Gubler) syndrome: ipsilateral nuclear VII palsy with contralateral motor hemiparesis
  Caudal tectal (Brissaud) syndrome: ipsilateral facial spasm with contralateral motor hemiparesis
  Caudal tectal (Foville) syndrome: ipsilateral hemiataxia and Horner's, contralateral hemiparesis

- Temporal lobe syndrome: contralateral homonymous upper quadrantanopia, jargon aphasia (dominant hemisphere), psychomotor epilepsy, uncinate fits, motor incoordination, amnesia (tumour, infarction, haemorrhage, trauma)

- Thalamic syndrome (Déjerine and Roussy): contralateral hemidysaesthesiae and hyperpathia with burning thalamic pain, hemiataxia, disordered stereognosis, choreoathetosis (infarction, haemorrhage, tumour)

- Weber's (cerebral peduncle) syndrome: ipsilateral oculomotor palsy and contralateral motor hemiparesis (infarction of middle cerebral peduncle).

PROCEDURES AND DIAGNOSIS IN NEUROLOGY

Doppler sonography of extracranial arteries supplying the brain
(Reproduced after Ries, F. Dopplersonographie der extrakraniellen Hirnarterien, in *Hirninfarkt*, (eds Hartman, A. and Wassmann, H.), Urban & Schwarzenberg, München, 1987.)

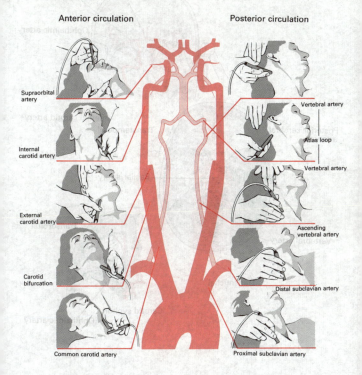

MEMORIX NEUROLOGY

Transcranial sonography

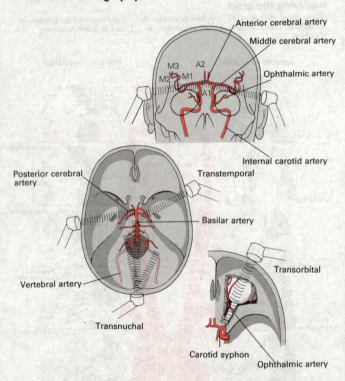

Identification criteria of intracranial arteries by transcranial Doppler sonography

(Reproduced after Ringelstein, E. *Noninvasive imaging of cerebrovascular disease*, (ed. Weinberger, J.), published by Alan R. Liss, New York, 1988.)

Artery	Approach	Insonation depth (mm)	Flow velocity (cm/s)	Flow direction	Other identification criteria
Middle cerebral	Transtemporal	50 (30–60)	55	Towards probe	Flow constant trace over 10 mm insonation depth
Anterior cerebral	Transtemporal	70 (60–75)	50	Away from probe	Flow reversal on common carotid compression
Carotid siphon (1)	Transtemporal	65 (60–70)	39	Mostly to probe	Relatively low flow
(2)	Transorbital	70 (65–80)	41	Mostly from probe	
Posterior cerebral (P1)	Transtemporal	70 (60–75)	39	Towards probe	Increased flow on common carotid compression
Top of basilar (P1 and P1′)	Transtemporal	75 (70–80)	39	Bidirectional	Demonstration of ipsi- and contralateral posterior cerebral artery
Basilar	Suboccipital	95 (70–125)	41	Away from probe	Change of flow on vertebral artery compression
Vertebral Extradural	Suboccipital	50 (40–55)	34	Towards probe	Lateral angulation of beam
Intradural	Suboccipital	70 (60–95)	39	Away from probe	Reduced flow on vertebral artery compression
Ophthalmic	Transorbital	45 (35–55)	21	Towards probe	
Internal carotid (extradural)	Submandibular	60 (35–80)	30	Away from probe	Insonation medially and posteriorly

Doppler sonography criteria for degree of carotid stenosis

(Reproduced after Hennerici, M., Neuerburg-Heusler, D. *Gefässdiagnostik mit Ultraschall*; published by Thieme, Stuttgart, 1988.)

	Non-stenosing plaque	Mild stenosis	Medium grade stenosis	Severe stenosis	Subtotal occlusion	Occlusion
Lumen reduction (%)	<40	40–60	60–70	about 80	>90	100
Indirect criteria	none	none	none	Inner canthus zero or retrograde flow Common carotid flow less than other side		
Direct criteria in stenosis region assessment						
Analogue pulse curve	NA	Abrupt flow increase	Marked flow rise, less pulsatility, systolic deceleration (turbulence)	Great flow increase, systolic deceleration	Variable stenosis signal with reduced intensity	Absence of vessel
Spectral wave form	NA	Broadening	Broadening, more low frequency components	Reduced, inverse frequency composition	Reduced, inverse frequency composition	Absence of vessel
Poststenotic findings	NA	NA	NA	Reduced systolic flow rate	Reduced: signal hard to find	Absence of signal
Systolic peak frequency of internal carotid artery (at 4 MHz pulsed Doppler)	<3 KHz	3–5 KHz	5–8 KHz	>8 KHz	Variable	Absent
Demonstrability by B mode imaging	Very good	Very good	Good	Moderate	Moderate	Moderate

NA: no abnormality detected

PROCEDURES AND DIAGNOSIS IN NEUROLOGY

Electroencephalography (EEG)
Diagnostic criteria of adult EEG at rest

Basic rhythms
(predominant activity)

Physiological: 8–12 Hz (Alpha rhythm) most marked in occipital leads
Disappears on eye opening
Reactivated by eye closure
Activated by hyperventilation
also
≥13 Hz (Beta rhythm) in frontocentral regions

Generalized abnormalities
(pathological basic rhythm)

Generalized slowing <8 Hz (Theta and/or Delta activity) geared to severity of disorder of function
Flattening of waves often linked to slowing as a feature of reduced cortical activity (burst suppression pattern)
Bursts of generalized rhythmic delta activity as a feature of subcortical dysfunction

Focal abnormalities

Focal slow activity (Theta or Delta focus)
Focal reduction of amplitude (flattening)
Increase in focal activity (e.g. focal epileptic discharges)
Phase reversal

Epileptic discharges

Steep transients (spikes and sharp waves) often in combination with slow after-discharges (slow waves) occurring focally or generally
Periodic epileptiform discharges lateralized or generalized in encephalitic illnesses, acute focal brain lesions or metabolic brain disorders

MEMORIX NEUROLOGY

Electrode positioning in 10–20 System

(Reproduced after Birnbauer, N. and Schmidt, R.F. *Biologische Psychologie*; published by Springer, Berlin, 1990.)

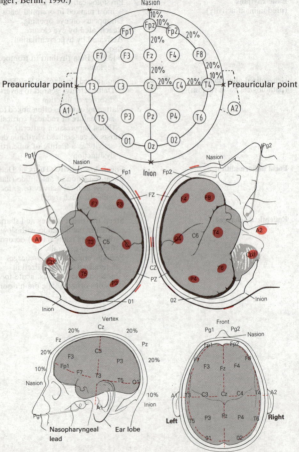

See also Jasper, H. (1958) *EEG Clinical Neurophysiology Journal*, **10**, 371–5.

EEG frequency bands
Frequency bands of the EEG

Alpha	8–13/s
Beta	>13/s
Theta	4–7.5/s
Delta	0.5–3.5/s

Statistical distribution of types of basic EEG rhythms
(Modified from Kubicki, S. and Höller, L. (1980) *EEG Laboratory*, **2**, 32–53.)

EEG basic rhythm	Total	Distribution by amplitude range			Heredity
		High (>50 µV)	Medium (10–50 µV)	Flat (<10 µV)	
Alpha (%)	86	5	77	5	Autosomal dominant
Beta (%)	7	–	3	4	Autosomal dominant
Theta (%)	6	–	1	4	Low voltage type: 9% (amplitudes up to 20 µV)
Mixed (%)	1	–	<1	<1	Autosomal dominant

Physical parameters for polygraph recording
(Modified from Höller, L. and Irrgang, U. (1981) *EEG Laboratory*, **3**, 65–82.)

	Filter		Amplification
	Upper limit (= time constant) (s)	Lower limit (Hz)	
EEG	0.3	70	50 µV = 7.0 mm
EMG	0.1	70	20 µV = 8.5 mm
EOG	0.3	70	50 µV = 7.0 mm
ECG	*1.0–1.5	70	*100 µV = 3.5–7.0 mm
Respiration	*1.0–5.0	30	50 µV = 7.0 mm

* Optional magnitude of upper limit filter and amplification

Variants of normal EEG

(Modified from Kubicki, S. and Holler, L. (1980) Systemization of basic EEG rhythms and normal variation. *EEG Laboratory*, **2**, 32–53.)

Variant	Heredity	Prevalence	Vigilance	Localization	Age
Occipital Theta variant	Autosomal recessive?	Different authors: 0.03–0.5%	Awake, relaxed, eyes closed	Occipital, posterior temporal, like alpha rhythm	Rarely before 6th year, declines with ageing
Mu waves	Not proven	Different authors: 2.8–57%	Awake, motor relaxation	Rolandic area (central region)	From 6th year onwards approximately
Beta groups	Autosomal dominant / Simply dominant	Type 1 0.45% / Type 2 1.47%	Awake and light sleep	Frontal and precentral	Preschool age
Lambda waves	Not proven	Age dependent 35.2–82.8%	Awake, visually active	Occipital (lambda region)	Mainly before 11th year
Positive occipital sharp transients of sleep	Not proven	49–79%	Sleep (NREM 1–3)	Occipital	Mainly after 16th year
Alpha sleep type	Not proven	15%	Sleep (NREM)	Frontal	Mainly after 16th year

Stages of sleep in the EEG

(Modified from Kugler, J. *Elekroencephalographie in Klinik und Praxis*, 3rd edn, published by Thieme, Stuttgart, 1981.)

Rechtschaffen and Kales	Dement and Kleitman	Loomis	Kugler	Demeanour	EEG Wave Pattern — Main feature	EEG Wave Pattern — Reactivity
W			A_0	Wakeful	Occipital alpha Normal variant	Visual blocking reaction (VBR)
NON-REM 1	I	A	A_1 A_2	Subvigilant	Diffuse alpha Alpha flat, sparse, slow Theta flat	VBR diminished VBR paradoxical
NON-REM 1		B	B_0 B_1 B_2	Drowsy	Theta flat Single alpha waves Theta flat to medium Theta medium height	VBR absent Flat vertex waves High vertex waves
NON-REM 2	II	C	C_0 C_1 C_2	Light sleep	High theta 30% of time High theta 50% of time High theta slow, continuous	K complexes
NON-REM 3	III	D	D_0 D_1 D_2	Medium sleep	Delta up to 30% of time Delta up to 50% of time Delta up to 80% of time	Broad K complexes Delta activation
NON-REM 4	IV	E	E	Deep sleep	Delta continuously	None
			F	Anaesthesia Coma	Periodic slow bursts, flat periods	None
REM	$\bar{V}$	REM	B/REM	Rapid eye movement periods	Low, fast, A_1–B_2 with eye movements	Partly none (B) Partly vertex waves

Brain mapping (EEG cartography)
(Reproduced after German EEG Society guidelines. Hermann, H. et al. (1989) *Zeitschrift EEG-EMG*, **20**, 125–32.)

Definition
Representation of spatial distribution of EEG potential measurements on the scalp by multichannel EEG leads or by evoked potential (EP) recording.

Data
EEG recording of at least 19 positions of 10–20 System and recording of eye artefacts (lateral and vertical):
1. 10 s after eye closure during 2nd and 3rd min of recording (2–20 s)
2. Immediately after eye opening, 2nd and 3rd min of recording (2–20 s)
3. At end of 3 min of hyperventilation (1–20 s).
(NB Concurrent visual checking of EEG recording for artefacts.)

Cartography
The base variable of the EEG is the mean amplitude (square root of performance per frequency band) for at least six frequency bands (0.5–3.4 Hz: 3.5–7.4 Hz: 7.5–12.4 Hz: 12.5–17.9 Hz: 18.0–fN: 0.5 Hz–fN (Nyquist frequency)).

The base variable for EP is the global latency within the chosen time window with localization of maxima and minima.

Display of interpolation algorithm and of linear scale of greyness or of colour scheme (black or red = high values or high differential; white or blue = low values or negative differential).

Display of amplitude chart from chosen time segment: mean amplitude of a frequency band (µV); or a potential chart: mean performance of a frequency band (µV).

Chart for one point in time for EP, spikes, K complexes (µV amplitude).

Analysis
Of data exclusively from actual recorded lead positions (no interpolated values): exploratory (p_e), descriptive (p_d) and confirmatory (p_k).

PROCEDURES AND DIAGNOSIS IN NEUROLOGY

EMG: procedural steps in conventional needle electrode myography

1. **Spontaneous activity**
   (a) **Physiological**
   Insertion activity
   End-plate rumble
   End-plate potentials
   Benign fasciculations

   (b) **Pathological**
   Fibrillation potentials
   Positive sharp waves
   Pseudomyotonic discharges
   (complex repetitive discharges)
   Fasciculations
   Myokymia
   Myotonic discharges
   Doublets, triplets, multiplets

2. **Motor action potentials**
   (formal descriptive characteristics)
   Duration
   Amplitude
   Phase (monophasic, biphasic, triphasic, tetraphasic, polyphasic)
   Polarity of phases
   Rise time (= steepness of potentials: normal 0.2–0.8 ms)
   Turns
   Satellites
   Blocking
   Recruitment factor $\dfrac{\text{Frequency}}{\text{Number of motor units}} = 5$

3. **Activity pattern**
   Single oscillations
   Reduced interference pattern
   Enhanced interfevence pattern

EMG patterns: constellations of normal, neuropathic and myopathic

(Reproduced from Neundorfer, B. *Polyneuritis and polyneuropathy*; published by V.C.H., Weinheim, 1987.)

	EMG findings Normal	Denervation	Myopathy
Insertional activity	Duration up to 300 ms	Increased	
Single motor unit potential	0.2–4 mV 5–12 ms	Recruitment reduced 2 mV or more 10 ms Increased, broader, Splintered polyphasic	200 μV 5 ms small, polyphasic, early recruitment
Spontaneous activity	—	fibrillations 100 μV 5 ms positive sharp waves	isolated or positive waves
Interference pattern	≥50 discharges/s (1–5 mv) 1 mV	Reduced high amplitude 1 mV	At weak contraction early full interference pattern, low amplitude 1 mV

Needle EMG of important muscles: normal findings

(Reproduced after Ludin, H.P. *Praktische Elektromyographie* 3rd edn; published by Enke, Stuttgart, 1988.)

Mean Potential Duration in ms

Age (Years)	Orbicularis oris	Deltoid	Biceps brachii	Abductor pollicis brevis	Abductor digiti minimi	Vastus lateralis	Tibialis anterior	Gastrocnemius
0	4.9	7.8	7.7	6.2	6.2	9.7	9.5	7.2
3	5.1	8.3	8.2	6.8	6.8	10.3	10.1	7.7
5	5.3	8.6	8.5	7.3	7.3	10.7	10.5	8.0
8	5.5	9.0	8.9	7.9	7.9	11.2	11.0	8.4
10	5.7	9.3	9.1	8.3	8.3	11.5	11.2	8.6
13	5.9	9.6	9.4	8.7	8.7	11.8	11.6	8.8
15	6.0	9.8	9.6	9.0	9.0	12.1	11.7	8.9
18	6.1	10.0	9.8	9.2	9.2	12.3	12.1	9.2
20	6.2	10.2	10.0	9.2	9.2	12.6	12.3	9.4
25	6.2	10.5	10.3	9.2	9.2	13.0	12.7	9.7
30	6.3	10.7	10.6	9.3	9.3	13.4	13.1	10.0
35	6.3	11.1	10.9	9.3	9.3	13.7	13.4	10.2
40	6.4	11.3	11.1	9.3	9.3	14.0	13.6	10.4
45	6.4	11.4	11.2	9.4	9.4	14.1	13.8	10.5
50	6.5	11.6	11.4	9.4	9.4	14.4	14.0	10.7
55	6.5	11.8	11.6	9.4	9.4	14.6	14.3	10.9
60	6.6	12.1	11.9	9.5	9.5	15.0	14.7	11.2
65	6.6	12.4	12.2	9.5	9.5	15.4	15.0	11.5
70	6.7	12.6	12.4	9.5	9.5	15.6	15.3	11.7
75	6.7	12.8	12.6	9.5	9.5	15.9	15.5	11.8
80	6.8	13.0	12.8	9.5	9.5	16.1	15.7	12.0

Nerve conduction velocity of median nerve

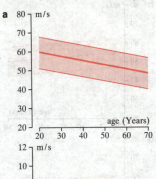

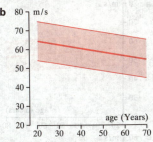

Median nerve: normal range of motor conduction velocities related to age (a) Elbow to wrist, $v_a = 64.482 - 0.23 \times age$, SD = 3.338; (b) arm to elbow, $v_b = 69.274 - 0.229 \times age$, SD = 5.729.

Median nerve: normal range of distal latencies related to age. Distances corrected for 6.5 cm. $t = 2.994 + 0.004 \times age$, SD = 0.392.

Nerve conduction velocity of tibial nerve

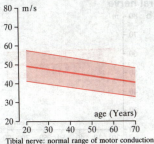

Tibial nerve: normal range of motor conduction velocity related to age between popliteal fossa and medial malleolus, $v = 53.697 - 0.166 \times age$, SD = 3.372.

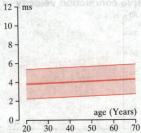

Tibial nerve: normal range of distal latencies related to age to abductor hallucis muscle on stimulation at medial malleolus. Distances corrected for 10 cm. $t = 4.021 \times age$, SD = 0.739.

Nerve conduction velocity of common peroneal nerve

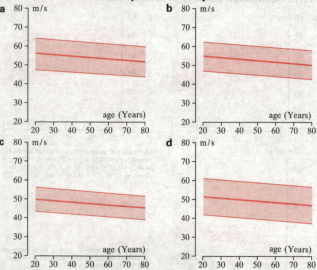

Common peroneal nerve: normal range of orthodromic motor and sensory conduction velocities related to age, after Singh *et al.* (1974). (a) and (b) sensory conduction velocity between ankle joint and distal head of fibula (a) and between distal head of fibula and popliteal fossa. (c) and (d) motor conduction velocities between head of fibula and ankle joint (c) and between popliteal fossa and distal head of fibula (d).

Nerve conduction velocity of sural nerve

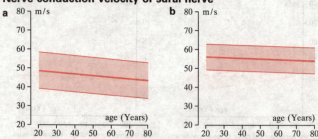

Sural nerve: normal range of sensory orthodromic conduction velocity related to age (a) dorsum of foot to lateral malleolus $v_a = 51.8 - 0.06 \times$ age, SD = 4.6. (b) lateral malleolus to midcalf $v_b = 57.4 - 0.04 \times$ age, SD = 3.7.

PROCEDURES AND DIAGNOSIS IN NEUROLOGY

Nerve conduction velocity of ulnar nerve

(Reproduced from Ludin, H.P. *Praktische Elektromyographie*, 3rd edn; published by Enke, Stuttgart, 1988.)

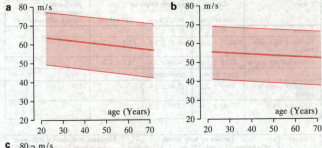

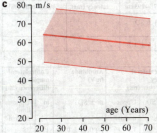

Ulnar nerve: normal range of motor conduction velocities related to age. (a) Distal ulnar groove to wrist, $v_a = 61.78 - 0.06 \times age$, SD = 7.58. (b) Proximal to distal ulnar groove $v_b = 55.63 - 0.03 \times age$, SD = 7.54. (c) Arm to proximal ulnar groove, $v_c = 64.39 - 0.1 \times age$, SD = 7.66.

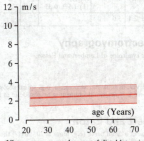

Ulnar nerve: normal range of distal latencies related to age. Distances corrected for 7 cm $t = 2.12 + 0.01 \times age$, SD = 0.34.

Normal range of F wave, H reflex and blink reflex

(Reproduced after Stöhr, M. and Bluthardt, M. *Atlas der klin. Elektromyographie and Neurographie*; Kohlhammer, Stuttgart, 1983.)

F wave	Latency (ms) by body length (m ± SD)			Maximum contralateral latency difference (ms)
	147–160 cm	163–178 cm	178–193 cm	
Soleus	29.48 ± 2.3	32.60 ± 2.1		
Extensor digitorum brevis	46.27 ± 3.2	49.32 ± 3.8	52.8 ± 4.2	
Flexor hallucis brevis	47.28 ± 3.6	50.60 ± 3.7	55.4 ± 4.2	
	from wrist	from elbow		
Abductor pollucis brevis	26.60 ± 2.2	22.40 ± 1.6		2.0
Abductor digiti minimi	27.00 ± 2.0	23.00 ± 1.6		2.0

H Reflex	Latency by body length			Maximum contralateral difference	
	147–160 cm	163–175 cm	178–193 cm	latency (ms)	Amplitude (%)
H reflex (soleus)	m ± SD	m ± SD	m ± SD		
	28.45 ± 1.8	29.9 ± 2.12	31.5 ± 1.2	2.2	50

Blink reflex	Latency (ms)		Contralateral latency difference (ms)		Amplitude (mV)		Contralateral amplitude difference (%)	
Orbicularis oculi reflex	m ± SD	Upper limit normal	m ± SD	Upper limit normal	m ± SD		m	Upper limit normal
R_1	11.4 ± 0.9	13.3 (14)	0.3 ± 0.6	1.3	(r) 0.73 ± 0.36 (1) 0.68 ± 0.29		19	38
R_2 (ipsilateral)	31.6 ± 3.2	38.1 (40)	0.3 ± 1.9	4.3 (5)	(r) 1.1 ± 0.39 (1) 1.1 ± 0.35		23	34
R_2 (contralateral)	32.4 ± 3.0	38.5 (40)	0.5 ± 2.1	5.0				

Repetitive nerve stimulation electromyography

Differentiation of myasthenia gravis and myasthenic syndrome of Lambert and Eaton.

Myasthenia gravis

On repetitive (3 Hz) supramaximal stimulation of nerves, as proximal as possible, e.g. spinal accessory nerve with EMG recording from trapezius mucle, there is typically a decrement in amplitude of at least 10% and no increment in amplitude.

Myasthenic syndrome of Lambert and Eaton

On high frequency supramaximal (tetanic) stimulation of a distal nerve (e.g. ulnar at 20–50 Hz) there is a characteristic increment of 100–400%. This is very painful, and a preferable screening test is nerve stimulation before and after 10s maximal contraction: in the myasthenic syndrome there may be a comparable increment. Normal people may show a maximum of 40–50% of facilitation.

PROCEDURES AND DIAGNOSIS IN NEUROLOGY

Latency ranges of evoked potentials

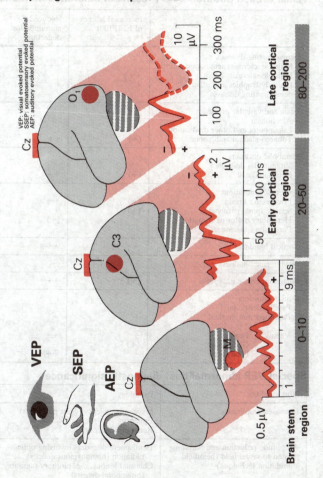

Visual evoked potential (VEP) results in different conditions

	Increased latency of P2 (P100)	Reduced amplitude/lost deflection

Demyelinating diseases
  Multiple sclerosis: acute optic neuritis
  Multiple sclerosis: latent
  Leucodystrophies and other demyelinating diseases
	
	+++
	+
		
		+++
		
		+

Toxic and vascular processes
  Alcoholism
  Ethambutol and other medication
  Tobacco-alcohol amblyopia
	
	(+)
		
		++

Metabolic disorders
  Vitamin B_{12} deficiency
  Neurolipidoses
	
	++
	(+)
		
		−
		++

System degenerations
  Friedreich's ataxia
  Spastic spinal paralysis
  Hereditary motor neuropathy
  Parkinson's disease
	
	(+)
	(+)
	−
	+
		
		++
		+
		(+)
		−

Cortical blindness	−	+++
Psychogenic blindness	−	−
Inflammations, e.g. syphilis	(+)	++

Ocular disorders
  Papilloedema: mild
  Papilloedema: marked
    ↕
  Versus Papillitis
             Glaucoma
             Panuveitis
	
	−
	+
	
	−
	(+)
	−
		
		−
		−
		
		++
		−
		+++

Special VEP abnormalities: diagnostic significance

Abnormalities	Pathology
Increased amplitudes	Myoclonic epilepsy (giant potentials) Epilepsy Renal insufficiency
Amplitude reduction and flattening related to visual field (hemifield stimulation technique)	Hemisphere disorders involving optic radiation (homonymous deficits) Chiasmal lesions, e.g. pituitary tumours (bitemporal deficits)

PROCEDURES AND DIAGNOSIS IN NEUROLOGY

Auditory evoked potentials (AEP): diagnostic criteria
(comparison of both sides is mandatory)

1. Loss/flattening of individual potentials (peaks)		I–VII
		I–VII
2. Absolute latencies of each peak		I–II
3. Interpeak latencies	IPL	I–III
		I–V
		III–V
4. Amplitude quotient V/I: normal > 1		

AEP: indication of site of lesion by peak drop-out
(Reproduced after Maurer, K. *et al. Evozierte Potentiale*; Ehke, Stuttgat, 1988.)

Normal pattern Preservation of peaks I–VII	
Midbrain disorder Loss of peaks VI/VII	
Pontomesencephalic junction disorder Peaks I–IV no abnormality Abnormal from peak V on	
Upper pontine disorder Peaks I–III no abnormality Abnormal from peak IV on	
Lower pontine disorder Peaks I and II no abnormality Abnormal from peak III on	
Disorder of VIII nerve (e.g. neurinoma) No potentials after peak I	
Cochlear disorder Loss of all potentials	

MEMORIX NEUROLOGY

Indications for use of Auditory Evoked Potentials (AEP) in diagnosis

Indication	Criteria/data
Objective determination of auditory threshold	Peak V
Monitoring of thrombolytic therapy in basilar occlusion	Delayed peaks II–V recover with successful treatment
Intraoperative monitoring (e.g. cerebellopontine angle tumours)	Latencies and amplitude changes of peaks II–V
Prognosis in coma (presupposes preservation of Peak I, by repeated assessments)	Poor prognostic data are absence of peaks VI/VII primarily, subsequently increased IPL (interpeak latency), craniocaudal loss of single peaks, development of desynchronization
Diagnosis of brain death	Sequential tests show craniocaudal loss of all peaks (on occasion peaks I and II may be preserved

NB Delayed latency of **p300** may be a neurophysiological parameter of various psychiatric illnesses (dementias, psychoses, etc.). It is only of minor use in the localization of neurological disorders

PROCEDURES AND DIAGNOSIS IN NEUROLOGY

Auditory pathways – AEP

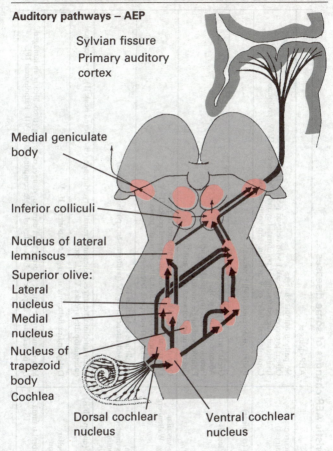

Anatomy of auditory pathways with sites of origin of potentials (Waves I–VII) (Reproduced after Spillmann, R. and Leitner, E. (1975) *Audiotechnology*, **24**, 11.)

Characteristic AEP changes of some diseases

Disease	AEP changes
Acoustic neuroma (Nerve deafness)	No pathognomonic changes Often: preservation of peak I with delayed peaks II–V Ipsilateral: ragged tracing of potentials beyond I, absence of IV/V, prolonged IPL I–V Contralateral: delay of V in brain stem compression
End-organ (cochlear) deafness	Ipsilateral absence of all potentials
Multiple sclerosis	Great variability of changes: Absence of single peaks Pathological IPL (interpeak latencies) Pathological single latencies Discrepancies between right and left
Brain stem vascular lesions (e.g. Wallenberg's syndrome)	Only dorsolateral lesions cause absence of peaks Unilateral/bilateral slowing of isolated peaks II–V Occasionally loss or flattening of single peaks II–V Pathological interpeak latencies
Alcoholism, Wernicke's disease, Central pontine myelinolysis	Amplitude reduction IV–V Delayed latencies IV–V (pontomesencephalic irritation)
Meningitis (encephalitis)	Often subclinical changes indicating cranial nerve damage (disordered peak II), or subcortical encephalopathy (peaks V, VI, etc.)
Spinocerebellar degeneration	Delay and/or flattening of single components II–V
Craniocerebral trauma	May demonstrate extent of brain stem damage, danger of coning (if cochlea is undamaged, i.e. preservation of peak I). Loss/delay of single components II–VII. Pathological IPL

Auditory evoked potentials (AEP): normal values

(Reproduced after Maurer, K. Akustisch evozierte Potentiale, in *Evozierte Potentiale* (eds Maurer, K. *et al.*), Enke, Stuttgart, 1988.)

Normal latencies (in ms) related to strength of stimulus (dBHL)

dB	x̄ SD	I	II	III	IV	V	IV/V
70		1.60	2.72	3.83	5.03	5.70	5.30
		0.12	0.19	0.20	0.21	0.22	0.25
80		1.50	2.65	3.73	4.97	5.60	5.20
		0.13	0.18	0.19	0.17	0.19	0.20
90		1.40	2.57	3.63	4.90	5.50	5.12
		0.10	0.14	0.16	0.15	0.18	0.18

Normal amplitudes (in nanovolt (nV)) related to strength of stimulus (dBHL)

dB	x̄ SD	I	II	III	IV	V	IV/V
70		220	180	250	280	300	430
		50	70	70	80	90	80
80		270	190	280	340	370	430
		80	100	100	90	90	90
90		290	210	290	350	390	450
		70	80	90	100	80	70

Normal interpeak latencies related to strength of stimulus

dB	x̄ SD	I–III	III–V	I–V
70		2.27	1.90	4.10
		0.15	0.18	0.15
80		2.29		4.10
		0.17		0.16
90		2.31		4.10
		0.13		0.16

MEMORIX NEUROLOGY

Somatosensory evoked potentials (SSEP): lead positions and response potentials

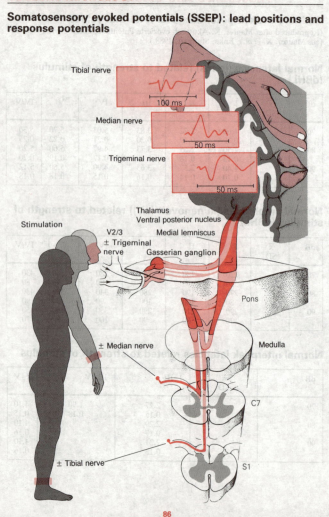

Positioning of leads for somatosensory potentials (SSEP) according to 10–20 Schema

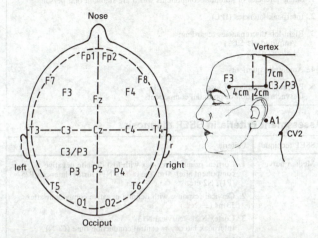

C3/P3 = C3' for median stimulation or P4' 2 cm behind Cz for tibial nerve stimulation
C5 (between C3 and T3) or C6 (between C4 and T4) for trigeminal stimulation

Common sites for stimulation and recording in SSEP diagnosis

Stimulus site	Recording site
Median nerve at wrist (motor and sensory nerve)	Brachial plexus (Erb's point) CV6 CV2 Contralateral cortical hand area C3' or C4' (postcentral gyrus)
Tibial nerve at medial malleolus (motor and sensory nerve)	Popliteal fossa LV5 (caudal) LV1 (lumbosacral response) CV6 Sensory cortex leg area Cz' (postcentral gyrus)
Trigeminal nerve (lip)	Contralateral postcentral region (C5/C6) in 10–20 Schema
Skin stimulation (purely sensory)	Appropriate sensory cortex area

Critical data in SSEP diagnosis in general

1. Single latencies of potential components which are stable in that person

2. Interpeak latencies (IPL)

3. Right-left discrepancies regarding:
   Amplitude (>50%)
   Latencies

4. Amplitude quotients

5. Potential flattening or loss
   Desynchronization of potential components

Assessment criteria in SSEP diagnosis

SSEP techique	Criteria
Median nerve	1. Cortical primary complex with first definite negative component after 20 ms ($\triangleq$ N20 or N1), further latencies P25 (P1), N2 etc. 2. Cervical response with definite negative component after 13 ms ($\triangleq$ N13) 3. Cortex N20 – cervical N13 Interpeak latency = central conduction time (CCN) 4. N20/N13 amplitude
Tibial nerve	1. Cortical primary complex with first clear positive component after 40 ms ($\triangleq$ P40), further latencies 2. Lumbosacral responses (LV1) after 22 ms (negative peak $\triangleq$ N22) 3. P40/N22 amplitude
Trigeminal nerve	1. Positive peak after 19 ms ($\triangleq$ P19) 2. Amplitude N13/P19

Pathophysiology of SSEP or impulse conduction by underlying disease

Demyelination	Axonal degeneration
SSEP latency delay SSEP loss by conduction block Discrete reduction of amplitudes	No change in latencies but progressive reduction in amplitudes leading on to loss of SSEP
Clinical paradigm: multiple sclerosis	Clinical paradigm: alcoholic neuropathy
NB Combined abnormalities occur frequently.	

Clinical significance of SSEP diagnosis

1. Recording from leads in different sites allows localization of disorders.
2. Assessment of long myelinated tracts and nerves (definition of process of demyelination).
3. Recording of clinically silent lesions in somatosensory system.
4. Objective proof of sensory symptoms.

Clinical applications of SSEP

- Disseminated encephalomyelitis
- Spinal disorders (e.g. space occupying lesions)
- Posterior column disorders: B_{12} deficiency
  Tabes dorsalis
  Friedreich's ataxia
- Cervical myelopathy
- Plexus lesions
- Radiculopathies
- Brain stem disorders
- Thalamic disorders
- Psychogenic sensory symptoms.

NB Dissociated sensory deficits (as, for instance, in cord vascular lesions) are not definable by SSEP.

Dynamic (serial) application of SSEP

1. In the course of monitoring of operations
   (a) Surgery for carotid artery stenosis
   (b) Surgery for correction of spinal scoliosis
   (c) Aneurysm surgery.
2. For prognostic assessment
   (a) Severe cerebrovascular accidents
   (b) Basilar artery thrombosis.

Common SSEP abnormalities in some clinical conditions

Clinical condition	SSEP abnormalities
Multiple sclerosis	Clear or even severe delay of cortical primary complex and of cervical responses, pathological right–left discrepancy of single latencies, pathological spinal and central conduction time
Posterior column disorders	Considerable amplitude reduction or loss, delay of single latencies, pathological spinal conduction time
Spinal space occuping lesion	Slight delay of down-stream lead potentials, reduction of amplitudes
Cervical myelopathy	Cervical responses poor or absent, slight delay of cortical SSEP
Brachial plexus lesion	Pathologically reduced quotient of plexus/N13 potential, occasionally delay of cervical responses
Thalamic disorders	Flattening, reduced amplitude up to loss of cortical primary complex (N20)
Huntington's chorea	Pathological flattening of cortical primary complexes (N20/P25 amplitude)
Epilepsy	Exaggerated cortical responses
Myoclonic epilepsy	Cortical giant potentials
Hemispheric lesions (infarct, tumour)	Unilateral loss or delay of single components of cortical primary complexes
Psychogenic sensory disorders	None

Prognostic significance of certain SSEP in severe cerebral disorders
(on peripheral median nerve stimulation)

SSEP findings (serial studies)	Prognosis
Complete bilateral loss of scalp SSEP (P15 + N20)	Very poor: survival unlikely
Severe deformation of scalp EP (only P15 detectable), or unilateral loss	Unfavourable: in case of survival, probable severe defect
Scalp SSEP preserved bilaterally with mild deformation of single potential components, or prolongation of central conduction time (N13–N20)	Survival probable, complete recovery dubious
Unremarkable scalp and neck SSEP	Generally good, probable complete recovery

SSEP in disorders of the spinal cord

(Reproduced after Jörg, J. *Rückenmarkserkrankungen*; published by V.C.H., Weinheim, 1992.)

1. **Spinal space occupying lesions**
   (a) Reduced cortical SEP amplitude, progressing to loss of deflection, mostly less delay than in multiple scherosis.
2. **Posterior column disorders**
   (a) Tabes dorsalis
   (b) Subacute combined degeneration of cord
   (c) Friedreich's ataxia
      (i) Considerable delay of cortical SEP, with reduction of amplitude
      (ii) Delayed spinal conduction.
3. **Cervical myelopathy**
   (a) Poorly defined SEP at CV2, possibly with normal SEP at CV6, frequently delay between CV6 and CV2 after median or ulnar nerve stimulation, possibly also delay between supraclavicular fossa (Erb's point) and CV6
   (b) Slightly delayed cortical-median SEP; occasionally absent, or reduced amplitude, SEP on tibial or peroneal nerve stimulation
   (c) Segment SEP with cervical or upper thoracic transection (loss of SEP, or reduced amplitude but very little delay of latency).
4. **Radiculopathies**
   (a) Segment SEP reduced or lost, with little N1/P1 delay (when two sides are compared)
   (b) Possible impulse conduction disturbance between supraclavicular fossa (Erb's point) and CV6, occasionally reduced CV6 SEP, rarely additional delay with normal N0 over CV6
   (c) Supraganglionic damage pattern with normal supraclavicular (Erb's point) SEP and normal N0 of the CV6 SEP with pathological N1 over CV6 (depending on site of lesion, on median or ulnar stimulation)
   (d) With lumbosacral root syndromes there is disordered conduction of SEP between popliteal fossa, or gluteal fold, or L5 and lead at L1
   (e) Pathological cauda equina recordings in L4–S1 syndromes (compare sides).
5. **Brachial plexus lesions**
   (a) Supraclavicular fossa (Erb's point) SEP delayed/reduced, or loss of SEP
   (b) CV6 SEP may show absent N0, occasionally with normal, or reduced amplitude, N1
   (c) In severe infraganglionic brachial plexus lesions there is loss of supraclavicular (Erb's point), CV6 and cortical SEP.

Median nerve SSEP at different levels (normal data)

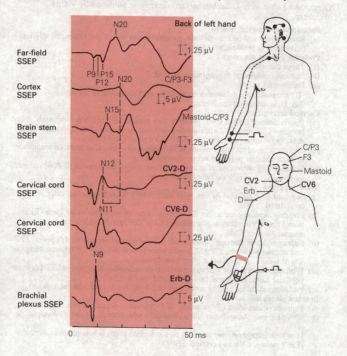

Normal data for SSEP from tibial nerve stimulation

(Reproduced after Riffel, B. *et al.* (1984) Spinal and cortical evoked potentials following stimulation of posterist tibial nerve. *Electroencephalography and Clinical Neurophysiology*, **58**, 400.)

Single latencies	N18 (L5)	N22 lumbosacral	N30 cervical	P40 cortical
Mean value ± 1 SD	18.4 ± 1.2	21.7 ± 1.6	29.5 ± 1.9	38.8 ± 2.0
Upper limit (mean + 2.5 SD)	21.4	25.8	34.3	43.9

Latency intervals	N18–N22	N22–N30	N30–P40	N22–P40
Upper limit (mean + 2.5 SD)	6.0	10.4	12.9	21.3

Amplitude quotients	N22–N18	P40/22		
Mean value (± SD)	3	4.9		
Scatter range	1.1–6.6	0.85–27.3		

NB In subjects above and below average height (<160 cm and >180 cm) values adjusted for body size must be used, particularly when cortical leads are recorded

Normal data for SSEP with trigeminal nerve stimulation

(Reproduced after Stöhr, M. and Petruch, F. (1979) SSEP following stimulation of trigeminal nerve in man. *Journal of Neurology*, **220**, 95.)

	Mean value ± SD	Upper limit (mean + 2.5 SD)
P19 latency (ms)	18.5 ± 1.5	22.3 ms
Amplitude N13–P19 (µV)	2.6 ± 1.0	

Magnetic stimulation: motor evoked potentials (MEP)

Principles
High energy magnetic fields (0.5–2.5 Tesla) are produced by brief current changes in a coil which in turn induce a current flow in the region of the neural structures for stimulation. It is feasible to stimulate cortical structures, nerve roots (e.g. C7, L3/L4), cranial nerves, plexuses and peripheral nerve, and to elicit a blink reflex.

Sites for stimulation
The illustration indicates sites for cortical stimulation of face, hand and leg muscles. Spinal stimulation of hand muscles is sited over the spinous processes C7/T1, for the leg muscles over L3/L4. Stimulation occurs at the intervertebral foramina. The spinal cord itself is virtually inexcitable by this method.

For cranial nerve stimulation the coil is placed ipsilaterally in a parieto-occipital position.

Advantages and disadvantages
1. A painless, non-invasive and rapid method of investigating central and peripheral motor tracts, and suitable for extensive routine application.
2. A supramaximal stimulus cannot be determined with certainty, and amplitudes must therefore be used in a limited way, particularly in stimulation of the peripheral nervous system. The exact site of stimulation of peripheral nerves cannot be predetermined.

Indications
Definition of the level of spinal and supraspinal disorders, demonstration of subclinical pyramidal tract lesions (particularly multiple sclerosis, motor neuron disease), exclusion of psychogenic 'paralysis'; the early diagnosis of idiopathic facial palsy.

Contraindications
Cardiac pacemakers, presence of ferromagnetic foreign bodies (particularly old aneurysm clips), severe cardiac arrhythmias, especially when cervical roots or brachial plexus are to be stimulated, epilepsy.

PROCEDURES AND DIAGNOSIS IN NEUROLOGY

Magnetic stimulation sites

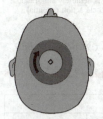 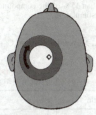 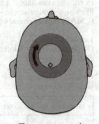

Target muscle
1st dorsal interosseous

Central stimulation
of facial muscles

Target muscle
Tibialis anterior

Transcranial stimulation showing various coil positions (marker at vertex). To stimulate thenar muscles a smaller stimulating coil must be moved contralaterally. When the coil is in a temporal position the physical current direction needs to be reversed. A frontal or parietal stimulus site may be used relative to the postvertex gyrus for stimulation of tibialis anterior.

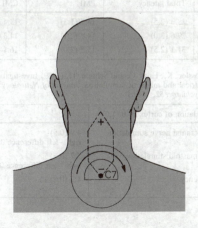

Anterior cervical roots are stimulated electrically with the cathode over C7. The centre of the coil is placed on the cranial side of C7.

MEMORIX NEUROLOGY

Magnetic stimulation: normal range

Amplitudes
In cortical stimulation a right–left discrepancy of over 50% is definitely abnormal, likewise a diminution to less than 15% of the compound muscle action potential (CMAP) on peripheral nerve stimulation.

Latencies
(Reproduced after Kloten, H., Meyer, B., Britton, C. *et al.* (1992) *Zeitschrift EEG EMG*, **23**, 29–36.)

CML/PML = central/peripheral motor latency in ms (standard deviation). Right – left discrepancies in excess of 2 ms are pathological

1st dorsal interosseous muscle			
Age	Total latency	PML	CML
19–29	20.6 (1.8)	14.0 (1.3)	5.8 (1.0)
30–59	20.7 (1.4)	14.6 (1.3)	6.0 (0.9)
>60	21.2 (1.6)	14.9 (1.4)	6.5 (1.1)

Tibialis anterior muscle			
Age	Total latency	PML	CML
19–29	28.3 (2.5)	14.7 (1.3)	13.4 (1.9)
30–59	29.6 (3.0)	14.7 (2.1)	14.3 (1.7)
>60	31.1 (2.5)	15.5 (2.0)	16.1 (1.9)

Nasal muscle (Rössler, K., Hess, C. and Schmid, U. (1989) Investigation of motor pathways by electrical and magnetic stimulation. *Journal of Neurology and Neurosurgical Psychiatry*, **52**, 1149.)

Magnetic stimulation of cortex 10.0 (1.0)	
Magnetic transcranial nerve stimulation	4.9 (0.5) right–left difference 0.3 (0.3)
Electrical stylomastoid stimulation	3.7 (0.5) right–left difference 0.3 (0.4)
Transosseal latency	1.2 (0.2)

Indications for lumbar puncture
(American Academy of Neurology (1993) *Neurology*, **43**, 626.)

Demonstration or exclusion of inflammatory processes
- Meningitis
- Encephalitis
- Polyradiculitis, polyneuritis, Guillain–Barré syndrome
- Multiple sclerosis
- Myelitis
- Vasculitides.

Confirmation or exclusion of subarachnoid haemorrhage

Confirmation or exclusion of a tumour with meningeal involvement
- Meningeal tumour infiltration
- Periventricular tumour.

Demonstration of specific antibodies in the CSF
- Tick-borne polyneuritis (Lyme disease, borrelioses)
- AIDS encephalopathies
- Neurosyphilis
- Para- and postinfectious polyneuritis

Beware of risk of causing a fatal coning by lumbar puncture in presence of raised intracranial pressure (suspicious history and/or papilloedema).

Cerebrospinal fluid (CSF)
Appearance at puncture
- Clear = Normal
- Turbid = Cell count $>300/mm^3$
- 'Purulent' = Cell count $>1000/mm^3$
- Xanthochromic = Old haemorrhage or very high protein, or severe jaundice
- Bloody = Recent haemorrhage: exclude 'traumatic' tap by collecting three serial samples and centrifuging – yellow supernatant fluid > 6 hours after haemorrhage

Normal CSF
- Cells: $0–5/mm^3$
- Total protein: 0.15–0.45 g/l
- Glucose: 48–70 mg/dl   about 50–60% of blood glucose sampled same time: 2.7–4.1 mmol/l   reduced in bacterial and fungal infections
- IgA: 1–6 mg/l
- IgG: 10–40 mg/l
- IgM: <1 mg/l

Common constellations of CSF abnormalities

Cells	Glucose	Protein	Other findings	Diagnosis
Polymorphopleocytosis > 300	↓	↑	Lactate ↑, possibly microorganisms	Bacterial meningitis, brain abscess
Mixed pleocytosis	↓	↑	Thread-like coagulum	Tuberculous meningitis, chemical meningitis
Mononuclear pleocytosis	Normal	(↑)	Possibly specific antibody changes	Viral meningitis or encephalitis
Mononuclear pleocytosis	↓	↑	–	Fungal, leptospiral, listerial or spirochaetal meningitis Recurrent benign (Mollaret's) meningitis Malignant meningitis
Mild mononuclear pleocytosis or normal	Normal	Normal	High IgG index	Multiple sclerosis
Normal	Normal	↑	–	Polyneuritis, Guillain–Barré syndrome

IgG index

$$\text{IgG index} = \frac{\text{CSF IgG : serum IgG}}{\text{CSF albumin : serum albumin}}$$

- IgG index <0.5: no evidence of intrathecal IgG production
- IgG index 0.5–0.75: intrathecal IgG production possibly raised
- IgG index >0.75: intrathecal IgG production is raised

(Oligoclonal bands: examine CSF and serum at the same time)

CSF changes in diseases of the nervous system

(Reproduced after Reiber, H. (1987) Liquordiagnostik. *Diagnosis Laboratorie*, **37**, 63–72.)

	Cells/μl			Activated B lymphocytes	Quotient albumin ×10^3†			Local Ab production Oligoclonal IgG	IgM	IgA	Specific Ab	Other
	n	<30	<300	>300		<10	<20	>20					
Purulent meningitis				X	X			X	(X)				Bacteria, neutrophils, CSF glucose ↓
Acute viral meningitis		X	X		X		X						Mononuclear cells
Fungal meningitis		X	X				X				(X)		Mononuclear cells, CSF glucose ↓
Tuberculous meningitis			X		X			X					Special stains, culture, glucose ↓
Tuberculous encephalitis	X						X		X				CSF glucose ↓
Herpes simplex encephalitis		X	X				X		(X)		X		PCR for early diagnosis
Varicella/zoster encephalitis	X						X		(X)			X	VZ virus antibody
Mumps meningo encephalitis		X							(X)	(X)	(X)	X	Mumps antibody
Measles meningoencephalitis		X										X	Measles antibody
Spring–summer meningoencephalitis	X						X		(X)	(X)		X	SSME antibody
Lyme disease	X				X			X	X	XX	X	X	Borrelia
Multiple sclerosis	X				X	X			X				Measles, rubella, VZ virus Ab
Chronic meningo-encephalitis	X				X		X		X				Endothelial cells: Mollaret's disease Epithelial cells: sarcoidosis Eosinophils: chemical meningitis
Neurosyphilis	X		X		X			X	X			X	TPHA
SSPE	X		X		X			X	X			X	Measles Ab
HIV encephalitis												X	HIV Ab

Data X apply to initial lumbar puncture CSF. (X) applies to follow-up CSF.
† Quotient albumin = CSF albumin/serum albumin.

CSF changes in diseases of the nervous system (continued)

(Reproduced after Reiber, H. (1987) Liquordiagnostik. *Diagnosis Laboratorie*, **37**, 63–72.)

	Cells/μl				Activated B lymphocytes	Quotient albumin ×10³†			Local Ab production Oligoclonal			Specific Ab	Other
	n	<30	<300	>300		<10	<20	>20	IgG	IgM	IgA		
Varicella-Zoster polyradiculitis	X				X							X	VZ virus Ab
Brain abscess			X										Mononuclear/ neutrophil cells
Parasitosis of CNS		X									X		Eosinophil cells
Guillain-Barré syndrome		X*				X							*In para-/postinfectious variant
Diabetic polyneuropathy							X						
Alcoholic polyneuropathy						X							raised glutamine in hepatic encephalopathy
SLE	X					X						X	Antinuclear Ab
Motor neuron disease	X					X							
Alzheimer's disease						X							
Haemorrhage						X	X						Erythrophages, siderophages
Brain infarct							X						
Primary brain tumour						X		X*					Neoplastic cells (CEA, α fetoprotein *with neuroma)
Malignant meningitis		X						X	X				Neoplastic cells (CEA), CSF glucose ↓
Non-Hodgkin's lymphoma													Neoplastic cells

Data X apply to initial lumbar puncture CSF. (X) applies to follow-up CSF.
† Quotient albumin = CSF albumin/serum albumin

PROCEDURES AND DIAGNOSIS IN NEUROLOGY

Blood tests in cerebrovascular disease

Full blood count

		Normal range	
Haematocrit (hct)	Females	35–47%	
	Males	40–52%	
Erythrocytes	Females	3.8–$5.2 \times 10^6/\mu l$	
	Males	4.4–$5.9 \times 10^6/\mu l$	
Haemoglobin (Hb)	Females	12–16 g/dl	<4.4–9.9 mmol/l
	Males	13–18 g/dl	8.1–11.2 mmol/l

Carboxyhaemoglobin < 1% (raised in CO poisoning), may be up in smokers.
Mean cell volume (**MCV**) 80–100: raised in alcoholism, liver disease, azathioprine treatment, B_{12} and folate deficiency

Coagulation

Partial thromboplastin time (PTT)	30–40 s
Plasma thrombin time	18–24 s (doubled or trebled when fully heparinized)
Thromboplastin time (Quick)	70–120% (10–20%: therapeutic range for oral anticoagulation)
Fibrinogen	200–450 mg/dl
Antithrombin III	70–100%
Plasminogen	80–120%

Vascular risk factors

Glucose (fasting)	70–100 mg/dl, up to 5.5 mmol/l	
HbA$_1$ (glycosylated Hb)	5–8% (indicator of mean glucose during last 2 months)	
Glucose tolerance test (75 g by mouth)	after 1 h <160 mg/dl, <8.8 mmol/l	
	after 2 h < 120 mg/dl, <6.6 mmol/l	
	after 3 h < 100 mg/dl, <5.5 mmol/l	
Insulin basal	5–24 µU/ml	58–172 pmol/l
Cholesterol	<240 mg/dl	<6.2 mmol/l
Triglyceride	<170 mg/dl	<1.8 mmol/l
HDL Females	>55 mg/dl	>1.42 mmol/l
Males	>45 mg/dl	>1.16 mmol/l

Blood tests in control of treatment for raised intracranial pressure

Osmolarity	285–295 mosmol/l

Blood tests in polyneuropathies

Tumour markers

Chorioembryonic antigen	<5 µg/l (bowel and thyroid carcinoma)
Calcitonin	<100 pg/ml (C-cell carcinoma, bronchial carcinoma)
Alpha-1-fetoprotein	<20 ng/ml (hepatocytic carcinoma, germ cell tumour)
Beta-2-microglobulin	up to 2.6 mg/dl (≤60 years)
	up to 3.1 mg/dl (>60 years)

Blood tests for poisoning

Lead	<400 µg/l	<1.9 µmol^3/l
Aluminium	14–37 µg/l	0.5–1.4 µmol/l
Thallium	0.05 µg/l	0.25 nmol/l
Mercury	<10 µg/l	<50 nmol/l
Manganese	<1.5 µg/l	9–27 nmol/l
Zinc	70–130 µg/l	10.7–19.5 µmol/l

Blood tests for vitamin deficiencies

Thiamine (B_1)	19–31 µg/l	56–92 nmol/l
Vitamin B_{12}	>130 ng/l	>96 pmol/l
Schilling's test	10–40% excretion in 24 h urine sample of oral radioactive marker B_{12}, preceded by intramuscular injection of unlabelled B_{12} 1 mg for saturation of plasma binding	
Folic acid	1.8–9.0 mg/l	4.1–20 nmol/l

Blood immunological tests for infections

Borrelia antibody (IFT)	≤1:220 U/ml (<1:4 in CSF)
Enterovirus Ab (KBR)	≤1:40
Epstein–Barr Ab (IFT-IgM)	up to (+)
Herpes simplex Ab (KBR)	≤1:160
Polio Ab (KBR)	≤1:10
Varicella-zoster Ab (KBR)	≤1:160
CMV Ab (KBR)	≤1:160
Mycoplasma Ab (KBR)	≤1:80
HIV	Negative

Blood test for Wilson's disease

Caeruloplasmin	18–45 mg/dl	58–145 IU/ml (low in Wilson's disease)
Copper	74–130 µg/dl	11.6–20.6 µmol/l

PROCEDURES AND DIAGNOSIS IN NEUROLOGY

Blood clotting

Clotting factors

Factor	Synonym	Comment
I	Fibrinogen	Soluble protein, fibrin precursor
II	Prothrombin	Alpha-1-globulin, proenzyme of thrombin
III	Tissue thromboplastin	Phospholipoprotein, acts in extrinsic system
IV	Calcium ions	Required for activation of most factors
V	Proaccelerin	Beta-globulin participates in prothrombin activation
VII	Proconvertin	Alpha-globulin, proenzyme, VIIa is protease
VIII	Antihaemophilic factor A	Congenital deficit: classical haemophilia
IX	Antihaemophilic factor B	Congenital deficit: haemophilia B (Christmas disease)
X	Stuart's factor	Alpha-1-globulin, proenzyme, Xa is protease
XI	PTA	(Plasma thromboplastin precursor)
XII	Hagemann's factor	Beta-globulin, proenzyme, XIIIa is protease
XIII	Fibrin stabilizing factor	Beta-globulin, XIIIa causes fibrin webbing

Clotting tests

Test	Normal	Test function/commentary
Platelet count	150 000–4 000 000/µl	Pathological result with thrombocytosis or thrombocytopenia
Thromboplastin time, TPT, Quick	14 s = 100%, Normal 70–120%	Global test of extrinsic system, assessment of coumarin treatment
Partial thromboplastin test, PTT	40–50 s	Global test of intrinsic system, assessment of coumarin treatment
Thrombin time, TT	17–25 s	Assessment of heparin treatment

For **therapeutic inhibition of clotting** the following anticoagulants are suitable:

1. **Heparin** occurs normally in the body, enhances action of antithrombin III, inactivates IIa, IX, X, thus inhibiting formation and action of thrombin. It needs to be given parenterally and has short duration of action (4–6 h). Antidote: protamine.

2. **Coumarins** e.g. warfarin, act as Vitamin K antagonists in the liver, thus inhibiting local synthesis of II (prothrombin), VII, IX, X: given orally, long acting. Antidote: vitamin K.

For **therapeutic fibrinolysis** the following fibrinolytic agents are available:

1. **Urokinase** promotes transformation of plasminogen to plasmin; antifibrinolytics have a reverse action.

2. **Streptokinase** derived from haemolytic streptococci, acts like urokinase and is equally effective in treating thromboses.

3. **Tissue plasminogen activator** (tpA) acts specifically on recent thrombi.

MEMORIX NEUROLOGY

Normal skull X-ray (semi-schematic)

(After Gerlach, J., Viehweger, G. and Pupp, J.S. Reproduced by kind permission of Boehringer Ingelheim.)

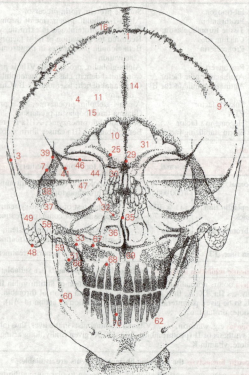

Front view

1. Sagittal suture
2. Coronal suture
3. Temporal suture
4. Lambdoid suture
5. Nasofrontal suture
6. Spheno-occipital synchondrosis*
7. Zygomaticofrontal suture
8. Wormian bone*
9. Diploic channels
10. Pineal gland calcification*
11. Choroid plexus calcification*
12. Ear lobe
13. Frontal bone inner table (thickened)
14. Falx calcification*
15. Frontal emissary vein*
16. Pacchionian granulation*
17. Sphenoparietal sulcus
18. Middle meningeal artery marking

PROCEDURES AND DIAGNOSIS IN NEUROLOGY

Normal skull X-ray (semi-schematic) (continued)
(After Gerlach, J., Viehweger, G. and Pupp, J.S. Reproduced by kind permission of Boehringer Ingelheim.)

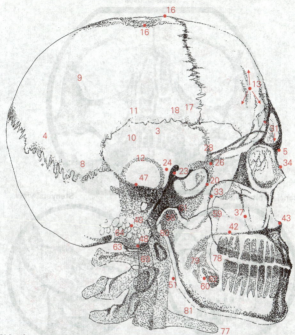

Side view
19 Occipital process*
20 Anterior margin of middle cranial fossa
21 Orbital roof
22 Floor of posterior fossa
23 Dorsum sellae
24 Calcification of tentorial insertion
25 Lesser wing of sphenoid
26 Planum sphenoidale
27 Clivus
28 Greater and lesser wing of sphenoid
29 Crista galli
30 Sphenoid sinus
31 Frontal sinus
32 Ethmoid air cells
33 Wall of maxillary sinus
34 Nasal bone
35 Nasal septum
36 Inferior nasal concha
37 Zygomatic bone
38 Frontosphenoid process of zygoma
39 Zygomatic process of frontal bone
40 Orbital margin
41 Linea innominata
42 Hard palate
43 Spine of maxilla
44 Superior orbital fissure
45 Optic canal
46 Lesser wing of sphenoid
47 Petrous temporal bone
48 Mastoid process
49 Mastoid air cells
50 External auditory meatus
51 Styloid process
52 Arcuate eminence
* Variable finding

MEMORIX NEUROLOGY

Normal skull X-ray (semi-schematic)

(After Gerlach, J., Viehweger, G. and Pupp, J.S. Reproduced by kind permission of Boehringer Ingelheim.)

Nasal sinuses

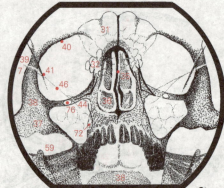

Optic canal (orbital) view

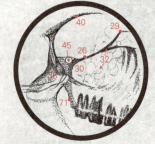

Stenvers' view

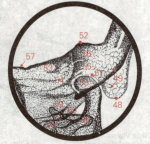

53 Internal auditory meatus and porus
54 Cochlea
55 Vestibule
56 Superior and lateral semicircular canal
57 Trigeminal impression
58 Head of mandible
59 Muscular process of mandible
60 Mandibular canal
61 Temporomandibular joint
62 Unerupted tooth*
63 Occipital condyle
64 Foramen magnum
65 Anterior arch of atlas
66 Transverse process of atlas
67 Atlantooccipital articulation
68 Lateral atlantomastoid articulation
69 Odontoid process (dens)
70 Bifid spinous process
71 Pterygoid process
72 Foramen rotundum
73 Foramen ovale
74 Foramen spinosum
75 Foramen lacerum
76 Infraorbital foramen
77 Hyoid bone with greater cornua
78 Tongue
79 Uvula
80 Ear lobe
81 Oropharynx
82 Trachea

PROCEDURES AND DIAGNOSIS IN NEUROLOGY

Principles of assessment of spinal X-rays
(Reproduced after Dihlmann, W. *Topographische Röntgendiagnostik III*; published by Thieme, Stuttgart, 1982.)

1. **Position and posture**
   (a) Segmental malposition
      (i) Posture in extension of segments (e.g. by muscle spasm)
      (ii) Dorsal gapping of intervertebral space
      (iii) Abnormal posture of several vertebrae above abnormal segment

   (b) Abnormal posture of part of spine
      (i) Thoracic kyphosis (increased or diminished)
      (ii) Lumbar lordosis
      (iii) Kyphosis of lumbar spine
      (iv) Scoliosis (describe deviation of vertebral axis by direction of convexity).

2. **Relations**
   (a) $\dfrac{\text{Vertebral body height}}{\text{Disc space}}$ = Dependent on age and disease

   (b) Normal disc space height:
      $C2 < C3 < C4 < C5 < C5 < C6 \geq C7$
      $L1 < L2 < L2 < L4 \geq L5$

   (c) Anterior dislocation

   (d) Posterior dislocation

   (e) Spondylolisthesis

   (f) Disc displacement

   (g) Alignment and intervals of spinous processes (contact between spinous processes with eburnation)

   (h) Size of transverse processes (L3 largest)

   (i) Psoas shadow (compare sides)

   (j) Paravertebral line

   (k) Anteroposterior diameter of canal (stenosis)

Principles of assessment of spinal X-rays (continued)

3. **Radiological morphology**
   (a) Shape of intervertebral foramina
       cervical: guttate; thoracic: ovoid; lumbar: auricle-like shape
       Anteroposterior projection of pedicles and transverse processes
   (b) Shape of vertebral body
       → Normal
       → Abnormal (total partial)
         → Uniformly: tall, flat, wedged, fish-like, box-like, cuboid vertebra
         → Unevenly
           — negatively: erosion, defect, infraction, decalcification
           — positively: distension, marginal osteophyte(s)
   (c) Vertebral structure
       → Normal (cortex, spongiosa)
       → 'Thinned' (osteoporosis, extreme 'ghost-like'), striped, thickened (sclerotic): circumscribed, circumferential, 'ivory' vertebrae, web-like, (poly)cystic osteolysis

Schema of important vertebral components in anteroposterior view

(Reproduced after Schinz, H.R. *et al.* Lehrbuch der Roentgendiagnostik III; published by Thieme, Stuttgart, 1979.)

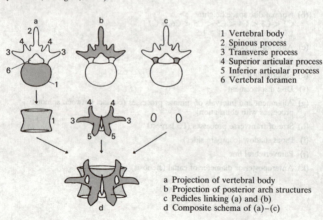

1 Vertebral body
2 Spinous process
3 Transverse process
4 Superior articular process
5 Inferior articular process
6 Vertebral foramen

a Projection of vertebral body
b Projection of posterior arch structures
c Pedicles linking (a) and (b)
d Composite schema of (a)–(c)

PROCEDURES AND DIAGNOSIS IN NEUROLOGY

Measurements for assessment of craniovertebral junction (X-rays)

Designation	Line joining	Normal
Chamberlain's line (1)	End of hard palate with posterior border of foramen magnum	Atlas and odontoid below line
Digastric line (2 a)	Mastoid notches	Odontoid tip below line
Bimastoid line (2 b)	Tips of mastoid processes	Crosses atlantooccipital joint; odontoid tip maximally 7 mm above line
McGregor's line (3)	Posterior margin of hard palate with lowermost point of occipital bone	Odontoid tip maximally 5 mm above line
McRae's line (4)	Anterior and posterior margin of foramen magnum	Odontoid tip below line

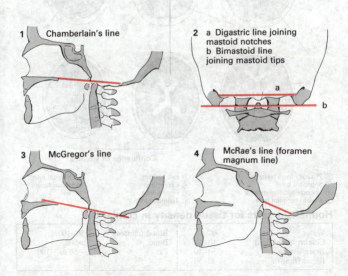

1 Chamberlain's line

2 a Digastric line joining mastoid notches
   b Bimastoid line joining mastoid tips

3 McGregor's line

4 McRae's line (foramen magnum line)

MEMORIX NEUROLOGY

Computerized tomography (CT) of head

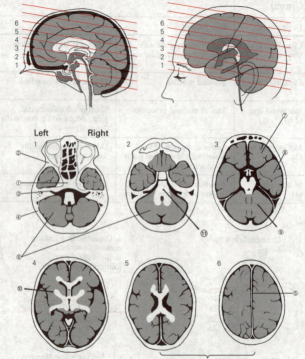

① Pituitary fossa (sella)
② Sphenoid bone
③ Internal auditory meatus
④ Parieto-occipital bones
⑤ Falx cerebri
⑥ Cerebellum
⑦ Frontal lobe
⑧ Temporal lobe
⑨ Occipital lobe
⑩ Sylvian fissure
⑪ Pons

Hounsfield units for tissue density in cranial CT

Water	0	Blood (clotted)	50–100
Cerebrospinal fluid	10	Bone	>500
Brain tissues	30–40	Fat	−50 to −100
Blood (fluid)	40–50		

PROCEDURES AND DIAGNOSIS IN NEUROLOGY

Density of lesions in CT of head

Hyperdense lesions
- Recent haemorrhage
- Calcification
- Bone
- Metastases
- Meningioma

Hypodense lesions
- Infarction (after 3rd day)
- Tumours
- Inflammatory foci
- Fat
- Air
- Old haemorrhage
- Cerebral oedema
- Post-traumatic changes

Isodense lesions
- Infarction (during first 3 days, in 2nd week, after contrast injection, depending on collateral circulation)
- Subacute haematoma
- Astrocytoma.

Effect of contrast injection on CT in common brain lesions

Enhancement after contrast	No contrast enhancement	Ring enhancement with contrast
Recent infarct Tumours, esp. metastases, gliomas, meningiomas Inflammatory foci Granulomas Angioma, aneurysm	Old infarct Old haemorrhage Demyelination Leucoencephalopathy Astrocytoma Behçet's disease	Glioma Brain abscess Metastases Subacute intracerebral haematoma Parasitoma

Calcification in CT of skull
- Oligodendroglioma
- Toxoplasmosis
- Calcified meningioma
- Fahr's syndrome
- Arteriovenous malformation
- Calcified aneurysm

MEMORIX NEUROLOGY

Anatomy of arteries of the brain

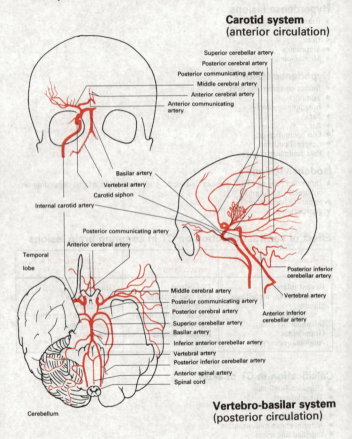

Planes of tomographic sections in magnetic resonance imaging (MRI)

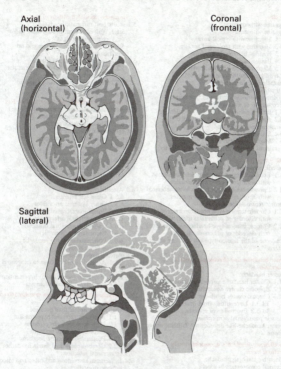

Axial (horizontal)

Coronal (frontal)

Sagittal (lateral)

T_1 vs T_2 weighted images

T1
- CSF: reduced signal intensity
- Fat: increased signal intensity relative to brain tissue.

  Appropriate for investigation of disorders of CSF circulation, foci of brain contusion, haemorrhages

T2
- CSF: increased signal intensity relative to cerebral tissue.

  Appropriate for demonstration of infarcts, inflammatory foci (including multiple sclerosis), tumours.

MEMORIX NEUROLOGY

Headache: classification
(International Headache Society of WHO (1988) *Cephalgia*, **8** (Suppl. 7).)

1. Migraine
1.1 Migraine without aura
1.2 Migraine with aura
 1.2.1 Migraine with typical aura
 1.2.2 Migraine with prolonged aura
 1.2.3 Familial hemiplegic migraine
 1.2.4 Basilar migraine
 1.2.5 Migraine aura without headache
 1.2.6 Migraine with acute onset aura
1.3 Ophthalmoplegic migraine
1.4 Retinal migraine
1.5 Childhood periodic syndromes that may be precursors to or associated with migraine
 1.5.1 Benign paroxysmal vertigo of childhood
 1.5.2 Alternating hemiplegia of childhood
1.6 Complications of migraine
 1.6.1 Status migrainosus
 1.6.2 Migrainous infarction
1.7 Migrainous disorder not fulfilling above criteria

2. Tension-type headache
2.1 Episodic tension-type headache
 2.1.1 Episodic tension-type headache associated with disorder of pericranial muscles
 2.1.2 Episodic tension-type headache unassociated with disorder of pericranial muscles
2.2 Chronic tension-type headache
 2.2.1 Chronic tension-type headache associated with disorder of pericranial muscles
 2.2.2 Chronic tension-type headache unassociated with disorder of pericranial muscles
2.3 Headache of the tension-type not fulfilling above criteria

3. Cluster headache and chronic paroxysmal hemicrania
3.1 Cluster headache
 3.1.1 Cluster headache periodicity undetermined
 3.1.2 Episodic cluster headache
 3.1.3 Chronic cluster headache
  3.1.3.1 Unremitting from onset
  3.1.3.2 Evolved from episodic
3.2 Chronic paroxysmal hemicrania
3.3 Cluster headache-like disorder not fulfilling above criteria

4. Miscellaneous headaches unassociated with structural lesion
4.1 Idiopathic stabbing headache
4.2 External compression headache
4.3 Cold stimulus headache
 4.3.1 External application of a cold stimulus
 4.3.2 Ingestion of a cold stimulus
4.4 Benign cough headache
4.5 Benign exertional headache
4.6 Headache associated with sexual activity
 4.6.1 Dull type
 4.6.2 Explosive type
 4.6.3 Postural type

5. Headache associated with head trauma
5.1 Acute post-traumatic headache
 5.1.1 With significant head trauma and/or confirmatory signs
 5.1.2 With minor head trauma and no confirmatory signs
5.2 Chronic post-traumatic headache
 5.2.1 With significant head trauma and/or confirmatory signs
 5.2.2 With minor head trauma and no confirmatory signs

6. Headache associated with vascular disorders
6.1 Acute ischaemic cerebrovascular disease
 6.1.1 Transient ischemic attack (TIA)
 6.1.2 Thromboembolic stroke
6.2 Intracranial haematoma
 6.2.1 Intracerebral haematoma
 6.2.2 Subdural haematoma
 6.2.3 Extradural haematoma
6.3 Subarachnoid haemorrhage
6.4 Unruptured vascular malformation
 6.4.1 Arteriovenous malformation
 6.4.2 Saccular aneurysm
6.5 Arteritis
 6.5.1 Giant cell arteritis
 6.5.2 Other systemic arteritides
 6.5.3 Primary intracranial arteritis
6.6 Carotid or vertebral artery pain
 6.6.1 Carotid or vertebral dissection
 6.6.2 Carotidynia (idiopathic)
 6.6.3 Postendarterectomy headache
6.7 Venous thrombosis
6.8 Arterial hypertension
 6.8.1 Acute pressor response to exogenous agent
 6.8.2 Phaeochromocytoma
 6.8.3 Malignant (accelerated) hypertension
 6.8.4 Pre-eclampsia and eclampsia

7. Headache associated with non-vascular intracranial disorder
7.1 High cerebrospinal fluid pressure
 7.1.1 Benign intracranial hypertension
 7.1.2 High pressure hydrocephalus
7.2 Low cerebrospinal fluid pressure
 7.2.1 Postlumbar puncture headache
 7.2.2 Cerebrospinal fluid fistula headache
7.3 Intracranial infection
7.4 Intracranial sarcoidosis and other non-infectious inflammatory diseases
7.5 Headache related to intrathecal injections
 7.5.1 Direct effect
 7.5.2 Due to chemical meningitis
7.6 Intracranial neoplasm
7.7 Headache associated with other intracranial disorder

HEADACHE

Headache: classification (continued)

8. Headache associated with substances or their withdrawal
8.1 Headache induced by acute substance use or exposure
  8.1.1 Nitrate/nitrite induced headache
  8.1.2 Monosodium glutamate induced headache
  8.1.3 Carbon monoxide induced headache
  8.1.4 Alcohol-induced headache
  8.1.5 Other substances
8.2 Headache induced by chronic substance use or exposure
  8.2.1 Ergotamine-induced headache
  8.2.2 Analgesics abuse headache
  8.2.3 Other substances
8.3 Headache from substance withdrawal (acute use)
  8.3.1 Alcohol withdrawal headache (hangover)
  8.3.2 Other substances
8.4 Headache from substance withdrawal (chronic use)
  8.4.1 Ergotamine withdrawal headache
  8.4.2 Caffeine withdrawal headache
  8.4.3 Narcotics abstinence headache
  8.4.4 Other substances
8.5 Headache associated with substances but with uncertain mechanism
  8.5.1 Birth control pills or oestrogens
  8.5.2 Other substances

9. Headache associated with non-cephalic infection
9.1 Viral infection
  9.1.1 Focal non-cephalic
  9.1.2 Systemic
9.2 Bacterial infection
  9.2.1 Focal non-cephalic
  9.2.2 Systemic (septicaemia)
9.3 Headache related to other infection

10. Headache associated with metabolic disorder
10.1 Hypoxia
  10.1.1 High altitude headache
  10.1.2 Hypoxic headache
  10.1.3 Sleep apnoea headache
10.2 Hypercapnia
10.3 Mixed hypoxia and hypercapnia
10.4 Hypoglycaemia
10.5 Dialysis
10.6 Headache related to other metabolic abnormality

11. Headache or facial pain associated with disorders of cranium, neck, eyes, ears, nose, sinuses, teeth, mouth or other facial or cranial structures
11.1 Cranial bone
11.2 Neck
  11.2.1 Cervical spine
  11.2.2 Retropharyngeal tendinitis
11.3 Eyes
  11.3.1 Acute glaucoma
  11.3.2 Refractive errors
  11.3.3 Heterophoria or heterotropia
11.4 Ears
11.5 Nose and sinuses
  11.5.1 Acute sinus headache
  11.5.2 Other diseases of nose or sinuses
11.6 Teeth, jaws and related structures
11.7 Temporomandibular joint disease

12. Cranial neuralgias, nerve trunk pain and deafferentation pain
12.1 Persistent (in contrast to tic-like) pain of cranial nerve origin
  12.1.1 Compression or distortion of cranial nerves and second or third cervical roots
  12.1.2 Demyelination of cranial nerves
    12.1.2.1 Optic neuritis (retrobulbar neuritis)
  12.1.3 Infarction of cranial nerves
    12.1.3.1 Diabetic neuritis
  12.1.4 Inflammation of cranial nerves
    12.1.4.1 Herpes zoster
    12.1.4.2 Chronic post-herpetic neuralgia
  12.1.5 Tolosa–Hunt syndrome
  12.1.6 Neck-tongue syndrome
  12.1.7 Other causes of persistent pain of cranial nerve origin
12.2 Trigeminal neuralgia
  12.2.1 Idiopathic trigeminal neuralgia
  12.2.2 Symptomatic trigeminal neuralgia
    12.2.2.1 Compression of trigeminal root or ganglion
    12.2.2.2 Central lesions
12.3 Glossopharyngeal neuralgia
  12.3.1 Idiopathic glossopharyngeal neuralgia
  12.3.2 Symptomatic glossopharyngeal neuralgia
12.4 Nervus intermedius neuralgia
12.5 Superior laryngeal neuralgia
12.6 Occipital neuralgia
12.7 Central causes of head and facial pain other than tic douloureux
  12.7.1 Anaesthesia dolorosa
  12.7.2 Thalamic pain
12.8 Facial pain not fulfilling criteria in groups 11 or 12

13. Headache not classifiable

Headache: differential diagnosis

Designation	Age at presentation and sex	Timing of onset	Localization and type of pain	Cocomitant symptoms	Triggers	Drug treatment
Migraine	Puberty, M < F, in childhood M > F	Onset often in morning may last 24–72 h, weekly recurrences	Hemicrania or unilateral start, mainly frontotemporal, changing sides, boring, throbbing, patient retires to bed	Nausea, vomiting, intolerance light and noise; possibly flickering scotoma, focal neurological symptoms	Some foods (cheese, chocolate), drinks (red wine), premenstrual, relaxation, alcohol, weather change	Beta-blockers, calcium antagonists, sumatriptan
Cluster headache (migrainous neuralgia)	Age 30–40 years, 80% males	Nights, often same time, 20–120 min. Daily for weeks, free for months	Unilateral periorbital, severe shooting pain, restless perambulation	Redness of eye and forehead, ipsilateral tear and nasal secretion, Horner's syndrome	None; occasionally alcohol, histamine, nitrate	Corticosteroids, serotonin antagonists, lithium, sumatriptan oxygen
Chronic paroxysmal hemicrania	Age 30–50 years, F > M	Day and night 5–30 min. No remissions	Unilateral, shooting, boring	Lacrimation, facial flushing and lid swelling	None; rarely head movement	Indomethacin
Trigeminal neuralgia	Older ages, more females	Numerous daily attacks, lasting seconds. Free months to years	Unilateral, mostly 2nd and 3rd division Unbearable, severe shooting, burning pain	Anorexia, avoids speaking, shaving triggering	Touching trigger points, chewing, swallowing, cold air	Carbamazepine, Phenytoin
Cranial arteritis	Over age 50 years	Day and night, continuous for weeks and months, no remission	Mainly temporal, dull pressure pain	Swollen tender temporal artery. High ESR. Possible visual disorder, joint and muscle aches (polymyalgia rheumatica)	Chewing aggravates ('claudication')	Corticosteroids
Tension headache	Adults, F > M	Waxes during day, lasts weeks	Diffuse, later worse at back, tight band	Insomnia, psychiatric symptoms, apprehension	Stress, psychological factors	Anxiolytics, antidepressants
Analgesics headache	Adults, 90% female	Morning–night, weeks, months	Diffuse, dull, pressing	Pallor, alopecia, anorexia, nausea, renal failure	Withdrawal of analgesic drugs	Beta-blockers, amitriptyline

HEADACHE

Differential diagnosis of cluster headache and chronic paroxysmal hemicrania

	Cluster headache (migrainous neuralgia)	Chronic paroxysmal hemicrania
Prevalence by sex	Male ≫ female	Female ≫ male
Age of affection	20–40 years	30–50 years
Site of pain	Orbitofrontal, strictly unilateral	Orbitofrontal, strictly unilateral
Accompaniments	Unilateral lachrimation and rhinorrhoea, conjunctival injection, Horner's syndrome	Unilateral lachrimation and rhinorrhoea, lid swelling
Course	Periods of pain lasting weeks, remissions lasting months, often worse spring and autumn	No remissions, daily attacks of pain
Diurnal pattern	Often at night, often at same time	None
Attack frequency	1–4/day	6–30/day
Attack duration	20–120 min	5–30 min
Triggers	Alcohol, GTN, histamine, certain foods	Rarely head movement
Treatment During attack Interval	Ergotamine, oxygen, sumatriptan corticosteroids, ACTH, serotonin antagonist (pizotifen), lithium	Indomethacin (aspirin)

Diagnostic criteria of drug-induced headache

1. Headaches > 20 days/month
2. >10 hours of headache per day
3. Drug use on >20 days/month (analgesics, ergot derivatives)
4. Headaches increase after cessation of drugs
5. No connection between continuous headache and pretreatment headache syndrome

Groups of drugs liable to cause headache

- Analgesics, anti-inflammatories, antimalarials
- Nitrate, antiarrhythmic agents
- Ergot derivatives
- Calcium antagonists
- Progestogens, oestrogens
- Benzodiazepines, barbiturates
- Muscle relaxants
- Corticosteroids
- Thyroid preparations
- Glycosides, diuretics
- Hypolipidaemic agents
- Various (acetazolamide, amantadine, bromocriptine, carbamazepine, griseofulvin, isoniazid, metronidazole, nitrofurantoin, phenytoin, rifampicin, theophylline)

MEMORIX NEUROLOGY

Pain localization in neuralgias of face and head

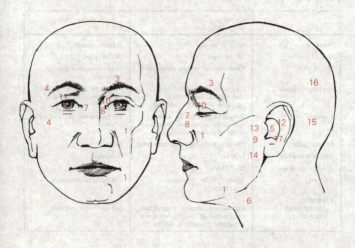

HEADACHE

Neuralgias and pain in face and head

1. **Trigeminal neuralgia:** commonly 2nd and 3rd divisions; attacks have trigger points (may be symptom of tumours, inflammation, Multiple Sclerosis)

2. **Anaesthesia dolorosa:** continuous trigeminal pain in hypalgesic or analgesic territory of nerve (after surgery or ophthalmic herpes zoster)

3. **Raeder's syndrome:** symptomatic neuralgia of 1st division with Horner's syndrome, possibly also ophthalmoplegia (middle cranial fossa pathology)

4. **Gradenigo's syndrome:** continuous 1st and 2nd division pain with disordered sensation, VI nerve palsy (tumour or inflammation in region of petrous apex)

5. **Glossopharyngeal neuralgia:** pain in root of tongue, throat, external auditory meatus (idiopathic, tumour)

6. **Neuralgia of superior laryngeal nerve:** laryngeal pain on swallowing, yawning, talking; with cough and hoarseness (infections, tumours)

7. **Nasociliary neuralgia:** paroxysmal orbital pain on touching medial canthus and chewing; associated with oedema and rhinorrhoea (idiopathic, infections)

8. **Neuralgia of sphenopalatine ganglion (Sluder's neuralgia):** minute-long attacks of pain in orbit, root of nose and upper jaw with lacrimation, rhinorrhoea and facial flushing (idiopathic in older females)

9. **Neuralgia of auriculotemporal nerve (gustatory sweating):** on eating a dragging pain with local flushing and sweating, lachrimation. Localized sensory disorder (after parotid surgery or parotitis)

10. **Vidian's neuralgia (greater superior petrosal nerve):** pain medial canthus (with tenderness), root of nose, upper jaw, palate, with sneezing (idiopathic, inflammatory)

11. **Tolosa–Hunt syndrome:** retro-orbital pain in superior orbital fissure syndrome (non-specific inflammatory)

12. **Geniculate ganglion neuralgia:** attacks of pain in the ear (vascular malformations, tumour)

13. **Costen's syndrome:** continuous facial pain in front of ear with burning in mouth, dizziness and tinnitus (anomalies of temporomandibular joint)

14. **Styloid process syndrome:** glossopharyngeal pain (from excessively long styloid process, local calcification or trauma)

15. **Occipital neuralgia:** paroxysmal pain along greater or lesser occipital nerve (idiopathic)

16. **Neck–tongue syndrome:** dullness and pain of tongue (lingual nerve) and of C2 on head rotation (compression of C2 root)

17. **Neuralgia of intermedius nerve:** deep ear pain, paroxysmal with trigger point in ear (idiopathic, varicella-zoster virus infection)

MEMORIX NEUROLOGY

Head and face pain: drug treatments

1. Migraine
   Beta-blockers: propanolol, metoprolol
   Calcium antagonists: nimodipine
   Serotonin antagonists: pizotifen, methysergide

2. Cluster headache (migrainous neuralgia)
   Corticosteroids, ACTH
   Lithium
   Methysergide

3. Chronic paroxysmal hemicrania
   Indomethacin

4. Tension headaches
   Amitriptyline, clomipramine, doxepin

5. Neuralgia (trigeminal, glossopharyngeal)
   Carbamazepine, phenytoin

6. Atypical facial pain
   Amitriptyline, thioridazine.

Migraine treatment

Treatment of acute attacks according to severity (and nausea/vomiting)

Aspirin	300–600 mg
Paracetamol	500 mg
Ergotamine	Orally 0.5–2 mg (maximum 4 mg/day)
	Suppository 2 mg (maximum 4 mg/day)
	Aerosol 0.36 mg, repeat after 5 min; maximum ×6/day

Additional antiemetic or psychotropic drugs as required.

Emergency treatment

Ergotamine tartrate	injection (s.c. or i.m.) 0.25–0.5 mg
Dihydroergotamine	injection (s.c. or i.m.) 1–2 mg
Sumatriptan	injection (s.c.) 6 mg, repeat once only after 1 h if pain recurs

Additional antiemetic or psychotropic treatment as required.

TUMOURS OF THE NERVOUS SYSTEM

Localization of tumours of the nervous system

Brain		Spinal cord
Supratentorial	Infratentorial	

Hemispheres
  Glioblastoma multiforme
  Astrocytoma
  Oligodendroglioma
  Meningioma
  Metastases
 	
Midline
  Pituitary tumours
  Pineal tumours
  Craniopharyngioma
	Adults
	  Acoustic neuroma
	  Metastases
	  Meningioma
	  Angioblastoma
	  (von Hippel–Lindau)
	
	Children
	  Cerebellar astrocytoma
	  Medulloblastoma
	  Ependymoma
	  Brain stem glioma
		Extradural
		  Metastases
		  Dermoid
		
		Intradural extramedullary
		  Meningioma
		  Neuroma
		  Angioma
		
		Intradural intramedullary
		  Ependymoma
		  Astrocytoma
		  Metastases

Treatment and follow-up recommendations for brain tumours in adults

(Reproduced after Krauseneck, P. (1986) Recommendations for treatment of brain tumours. *Deutsch Aerztebl*, **83**, 686–9 (in German).)

CT check 4 weeks after surgery provides a base-line for follow-up. In uncomplicated cases the following guidelines apply as regards timing:

1. Benign brain tumours (WHO grade 1)

   Follow-up examinations after 3, 6 and 12 months, always with CT, thereafter only if symptomatic.

   Pituitary adenomas require regular endocrine reassessment.

   In case of recurrence re-operation, possibly linked with, or replaced by, radiotherapy (e.g. craniopharyngiomas).

2. Semi-benign brain tumours (WHO grade 2)

   Clinical follow-up examinations with CT 3-monthly for a year, then at least once a year.

   In case of recurrence re-operation linked with, or replaced by, targeted tumour radiotherapy (tumour dose 60 Gy).

3. Malignant brain tumours (WHO grades 3 and 4, metastases)

   Radiotherapy at tumour dose 60 Gy, possibly chemotherapy for gliomas, ependymomas and medulloblastomas, possibly additional intrathecal treatment or prophylaxis.

   For metastases whole brain irradiation (30–40 Gy) and/or cytostatic chemotherapy (used primarily for meningeal tumour infiltration); cranial plus spinal irradiation for meningeal infiltration. Some neoplasms require irradiation only at first, but then CSF checks and possibly intrathecal cytostatic chemotherapy.

Brain tumours: indications for radiotherapy and cytostatic chemotherapy

Radiotherapy (50–60 Gy during 7 weeks)
- Malignant glioma
- Oligodendroglioma (after only subtotal surgical removal or if anaplastic)
- Dysgerminoma*
- Primary CNS lymphoma*
- Medulloblastoma**
- Ependymoma**
- Meningioma (malignant, inoperable)
- Pituitary adenoma (after subtotal surgical removal and after failed drug treatment)
- chordoma of skull base

* Primary radiotherapy (after biopsy confirmation).
** Prophylactic irradiation of skull and spine (40 Gy to each).

Chemotherapy
- Malignant glioma: BCNU intravenously (in selected cases)
- Primary CNS lymphoma: methotrexate (MTX) + cytosine-arabinoside (ArA C) intrathecally (Ommaya reservoir); alternatively irradiation of craniospinal axis
- Meningeal tumour infiltration: MTX + ArA C intrathecally, plus craniospinal irradiation

Karnofsky scale for disability grading in neoplastic disease

(Reproduced after Karnofsky, D.A. *et al.* (1948) *Cancer*, **1**, 634.)
100% – normal
90% – minor signs, normal activities
80% – normal life possible with effort
70% – cares for self
60% – cares for self with occasional assistance
50% – requires frequent care and considerable assistance
40% – disabled, requires special care (at home)
30% – severely disabled, hospitalized
20% – very sick, hospitalized
10% – moribund.

TUMOURS OF THE NERVOUS SYSTEM

Brain tumours: localization

Localization	Symptomatology	Tumour types
Frontal lobe	Personality change, headache Epilepsy (liability to serial fits) Hyposmia/anosmia	Meningioma (olfactory groove, sphenoid wing, parasagittal) Astrocytoma, glioblastoma, oligodendroglioma Metastases (bronchus, breast, melanoma)
Temporal lobe	Epilepsy (psychomotor attacks) Hemiparesis, aphasia, homonymous hemianopia, Personality change	Meningioma (sphenoid), glioblastoma, astrocytoma, oligodendroglioma Metastases (renal, gastrointestinal)
Parietal lobe	Epilepsy, hemiparesis, hemianopia	Meningioma (falx, convexity), glioblastoma, oligodendroglioma metastases (bronchus, breast, renal, melanoma)
Occipital lobe	Homonymous visual field defects, visual symptoms	Meningioma (parasagittal, tentorial), glioblastoma, metastases (bronchial, renal, breast)
Ventricular	Raised intracranial pressure (ICP) crises (obstructive hydrocephalus)	Ependymoma, plexus papilloma, epidermoid, dermoid, meningioma (falx), colloid cyst
Basal ganglia	Hemiparesis, thalamic syndrome	Astrocytoma, oligodendroglioma, glioblastoma, metastases (bronchus, breast)
Midbrain	Endocrine disorders (hypothalamus) Parinaud's syndrome, cranial nerve palsies, obstructive hydrocephalus (raised ICP)	Glioma (in children), pinealoma
Brain stem	Cranial nerve palsies, pareses, sensory deficits, raised ICP signs (obstructive hydrocephalus)	Glioma (in children), astrocytoma, metastases (breast, bronchus, renal), hypoglossal neuroma, clivus tumour (chordoma, meningioma, epidermoid, chondroma)
Cerebellum	Hemiataxia, tilt, hypotonia, raised ICP crises (acute brain herniation)	Spongioblastoma and medulloblastoma in children, 4th ventricle ependymoma, angioblastoma, metastases (gastrointestinal tract, bronchus, breast)
Cerebellopontine angle	Tinnitus, deafness, VII and V nerve compression, hemiataxia, headache; late: raised ICP	Acoustic neuroma, meningioma, dermoid, epidermoid, trigeminal neuroma
Sellar region	Headache, endocrine symptoms, bitemporal hemianopia	Pituitary adenoma, craniopharyngioma, meningioma (tuberculum sellae) epidermoid, aneurysm, optic nerve glioma in children

Types of brain herniation with raised intracranial pressure (ICP)

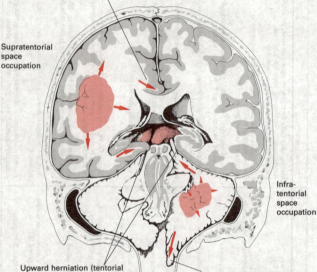

Midline shift under the falx may rarely lead to anterior cerebral artery occlusion

Supratentorial space occupation

Infra-tentorial space occupation

Upward herniation (tentorial herniation) produces disordered consciousness, ipsilateral pupil dilatation by III nerve compresion, eventually ipsilateral hemiparesis and extensor spasms

Downward herniation (tonsillar herniation) causes reactive neck – shoulder symptoms, disordered consciousness, circulatory and respiratory disorders, and extensor spasms

TUMOURS OF THE NERVOUS SYSTEM

Histological classification of tumours of the nervous system
(Modified for Kleinhaus, P. *et al.* (eds) (1988) *Tumoren des Nervensystem*, Springer, Berlin.)

Designation	Localization	WHO grade
Neuroepithelial tumours		
Astrocytoma		
Pilocytic	Cerebellum, optic nerve (childhood)	1
Fibrillary	Cerebral hemispheres	2
Protoplasmic	Cerebral hemispheres	2
Gemistocytic	Cerebral hemispheres	2
Anaplastic	Cerebral hemispheres	3, rarely metastasises
Giant cell	Subependymal, lateral ventricle (in tuberous sclerosis)	1
Oligodendroglioma		
Anaplastic	Cerebral hemispheres (frontal, basal ganglia)	3, CSF metastases
Isomorphic	Cerebral hemispheres (frontal, basal ganglia	2
Oligoastrocytoma	Cerebral hemispheres	2–3
Glioblastoma		
Glioblastoma multiforme	Cerebral hemispheres, corpus callosum (butterfly glioma)	4, CSF metastases
Gliomatosis	Cerebral hemispheres, brainstem, cerebellum	4
Ependymoma and plexus papilloma		
Ependymoma	Ventricles, sp.cord, cauda equina	1–2
Anaplastic ependymoma	Periventricular	3, metastasises
Papillary ependymoma	4th ventricle, cerebello-pontine angle	1–2
Myxopapillary ependymoma	Cauda equina	1–2
Subependymoma	4th ventricle, lateral ventricles	1
Plexus papilloma	Lateral & 4th ventricle (childhood)	1, CSF metastases
Anaplastic papilloma	Lateral & 4th ventricle	3–4, CSF metastases
Neuronal tumour		
Gangliocytoma	Central, temporal, 3rd ventricle adrenal (juvenile)	1
Ganglioglioma	Temporal, central, 3rd ventricle	1–4
Neuroblastoma	Sympathetic, hemispheres (childhood)	3
Olfactory neuroblastoma	Nasal cavity, sinuses (juveniles)	3, metastasises
Retinoblastoma	Eye (infants)	3, metastasises
Pineal tumour		
Pineocytoma	Quadrigeminal plate, aqueduct	1–3, CSF metastases
Pineoblastoma	Quadrigeminal plate, aqueduct (children)	4, CSF metastases
Embryonic tumours		
Medulloblastoma	Cerebellar vermis, 4th ventricle (childhood)	4, CSF metastases
Desmoplastic 11	Cerebellar hemispheres (juveniles)	4
Peripheral nerve tumours		
Neuroma	8th nerve, spinal nerves (posterior roots)	1
Anaplastic neurinoma	in neurofibromatosis	3, metastases
Neurofibroma	in neurofibromatosis	1
Anaplastic neurinoma	in neurofibromatosis	3–4

Histological classification of tumours of the nervous system
(Continued)

(Modified for Kleinhues, P. *et al.* (eds) (1988) *Tumoren des Nervensystem*, Springer, Berlin.)

Designation	Localization	WHO grade
Meningeal tumours		
Meningioma	Intracranial, extracerebral, spinal	
Meningotheliomatory	Falx, sphenoid, olfactory groove, tentorium, parasagittal, vault	1
Fibroblastic	Spinal (mainly women)	1
Angiomatous		1
Haemangiopericytic		2
Papillary		2–3
Anaplastic		3, metastases
Meningeal sarcoma		
Fibrosarcoma	Dura (children, juveniles)	3–4
Sarcomatosis	Spinal subarachnoid space (children, juveniles)	3–4
Primary melanotic tumour		
Meningeal melanoma	Intracranial or spinal	3
Neurocutaneous melanosis	Phakomatosis (congenital, infants)	2–3
Vascular tumour		
Haemangioblastoma	Cerebellum, spinal cord brainstem	1
Primary malignant lymphoma		
Malignant lymphoma	Cerebral hemispheres (periventricular)	3
Germinal cell tumour		
Germinoma	Pineal region, suprasellar (children)	2–3
Teratoma	Pineal region, suprasellar, spinal (children, juveniles)	1–3
Mixed germinal cell tumour		
Embryonic carcinoma	Intracerebral near midline	4
Choriocarcinoma	Intracerebral near midline	4
Endodermal sinus tumour	Intracerebral near midline	4
Malformation tumours and cysts		
Craniopharyngioma	Suprasellar (children, juveniles)	1
Granular cell tumour	Infra- or supra-sellar, extracerebral	1
Dermoid	Spinal (lumbosacral), posterior fossa	1
Epidermoid	Cerebellopontine angle, temporal	1
Lipoma	Corpus callosum, hypothalamus, quadrigeminal plate region	1
Colloid cyst	3rd ventricle	1
Rathke's pouch cyst	Intrasellar	1
Enterogenous cyst	Intraspinal intradural	1
Ependymoma cyst	Lateral ventricle, spinal	1
Neuroglial cyst	Brain, spinal cord	1
Arachnoid cyst	Sylvian fissure, posterior fossa	1
Tumours of adjacent structures		
Paraganglioma	Carotid body, glomus jugulare, cauda equina	2–3, metastases
Chordoma	Clivus, sacrum	1
Histiocytosis X	Skull, vertebral body	1
Hand–Schüller–Christian	(children)	
Letterer–Siwe disease	(babies)	
Eosinophilic granuloma	(juveniles)	
Metastases		
Metastases from bronchial carcinoma, breast carcinoma, melanoma, gastrointestinal tract carcinoma CSF-borne metastases from medulloblastoma, pineoblastoma, germinoma. Carcinomatous, sarcomatous and leukaemic meningitis		

TUMOURS OF THE NERVOUS SYSTEM

Hydrocephalus: differential diagnosis

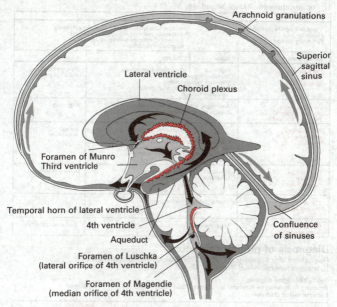

Pathogenesis	Anatomical site	Aetiology	Terminology
Blocked circulation	Foramen of Munro	Ventricle ependymoma, colloid cyst, ventriculitis	Obstructive hydrocephalus
	3rd ventricle	Ependymoma, plexus papilloma	
	Aqueduct	Stenosis, tumour	
	4th ventricle (foramina of Luschka & Magendie)	Medulloblastoma, craniovertebral anomaly, inflammation, subarachnoid haemorrhage	
Impaired CSF absorption	Arachnoid granulations, subarachnoid space	After subarachnoid haemorrhage, meningitis	Communicating or malabsorptive hydrocephalus
Increased CSF production	Choroid plexus	Inflammation, plexus papilloma	Hypersecretory hydrocephalus
Brain shrinkage	Local or generalized brain atrophy	Alzheimer's, Pick's disease, agenesis of corpus callosum	Compensatory hydrocephalus

Pituitary tumours: symptoms and signs
(Reproduced after von der Mühlen, A. (1989) Klinische Symptomatik bei Hypophysentumore. *Aktuel Neurol*, **16**, 38–42.)

General features	
Visual field defects (bitemporal) Headache Personality changes	Cavernous sinus syndrome (with parasellar extension) Hypothalamic features (with upward extension): disorders of wakefulness/sleep, of appetite & temperature regulation

Specific features	Males	Females	Children
Hormone secreting tumours (chromophobe)	Impotence Secondary hypoadrenalism Secondary hypothyroidism Diabetes insipidus (secondary posterior pituitary failure)	Secondary amenorrhoea	Pituitary dwarfism Failure of puberty
Growth hormone secreting adenoma (acidophil, eosinophil)	Acromegaly with visceral hypertrophy, diabetes and intestinal polyposis		Gigantism
ACTH secreting adenoma (mucoid, basophilic cells)	Cushing's disease: trunk obesity, striae, moon face, osteoporosis, hypertension, diabetes mellitus, thromboses, affective disorders	Hirsutism, menstrual disorders	Growth retardation
Prolactinoma (oncocytic, chromophobe)	Impotence Gynaecomastia	Secondary amenorrhoea galactorrhoea, impaired libido	Delayed puberty
TSH secreting adenoma (mucoid, basophilic cells)	Pituitary hyperthyroidism (very rare)		
Gonadotrophin secreting adenoma	Hypergonadism (very rare)		Precocious puberty

Diagnosis of pituitary tumours
(Reproduced after Schürmeyer, T. *et al.* (1989) Endokrinologische Diagnostik bei Hypophysentumoren. *Aktuel Neurol*, **16**. 43–45.)

Ophthalmological diagnosis
Perimetry to demonstrate symmetrical bitemporal field defect (upper quadrant → hemianpia)
Endocrinological diagnosis

	Normal	Definitely abnormal
GH level basal and after 100 g oral glucose	<1 ng/ml	>20 ng/ml
Cortisol in 24 h urine	<75 µg/24 h	>150 µ/24h
Dexamethasone suppression test (plasma cortisol after 2 mg dexamethasone)	<5 µg/dl	
Prolactin basal level	<20 ng/ml	>150 ng/ml
T3 and T4	T3 0.9–1.9 µg/l T4 45–130 µg/l	>150 µg/24h
Serum cortisol level		
Testosterone in men	>5 µg/dl	
Oestradiol in women	>3.0 ng/ml >40 ng/ml	

Occasionally need for stimulation tests with TRH, LHRH and GHRH

Neuroradiological diagnosis
Plain X-rays of skull (anteroposterior and lateral, coned view of sella)
Computerized tomography, without and with contrast enhancement
Magnetic resonance imaging (T1 and T2 weighting)
Digital subtraction arteriography (to exclude carotid aneurysm).

TUMOURS OF THE NERVOUS SYSTEM

Pituitary hormones: posterior lobe (neurohypophysis)

Formation and storage of ADH and oxytocin
(Reproduced after Wurtke, K. (1990) Endokrinologie, in *Physiologie des Menschen*, 24th edn, (eds Schmidt, R.F. and Thews, G.), Springer, Heidelberg.)

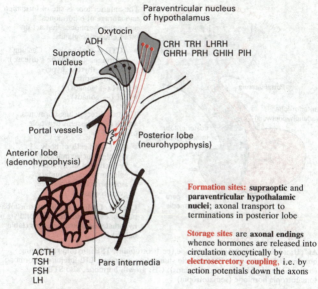

Formation sites: **supraoptic** and **paraventricular hypothalamic nuclei**; axonal transport to terminations in posterior lobe

Storage sites are **axonal endings** whence hormones are released into circulation exocytically by **electrosecretory coupling**, i.e. by action potentials down the axons

Actions of ADH and oxytocin

hormone	action – commentary
ADH	**Antidiuretic action:** stimulated by blood hyperosmolarity, inhibited by hypoosmolarity; release of ADH increases permeability for water of collecting tubules and distal convolutions thus causing antidiuresis (deficiency = diabetes insipidus)
	Vasopressor action: arterial vasoconstriction (raised blood pressure); severe fall of blood pressure (shock, haemorrhage) causes release of ADH with resultant rise in pressure
Oxytocin	**Milk ejection reflex**
	Labour induced at end of pregnancy (Ferguson reflex)

MEMORIX NEUROLOGY

Pituitary hormones: anterior lobe (adenohypophysis)

The four messenger and the two direct acting hormones of the anterior lobe
(Reproduced after Wurtke, K. (1990) Endokrinologie, in *Physiologie des Menschen*, 24th edn, (eds Schmidt, R.F. and Thews, G.), Springer, Heidelberg.)

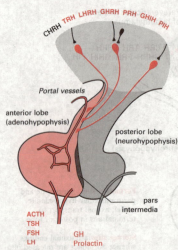

The anterior lobe is site of **formation and storage** of 6 hormones: 4 messenger hormones that act on other endocrine glands:

- **ACTH** (→ adrenals: ↑ Cushing's syndrome, ↓ Addison's disease)
- **TSH** (→ thyroid: hyper-, hypothyroidism)
- **FSH** (→ gonads)
- **LH** (→ gonads)

The two direct acting hormones act on other systems or whole organism:

- **GH** (→ all cells of body: ↑ gigantism or acromegaly)
- **Prolactin** (→ many cells: ↑ galactorrhoea, secondary amenorrhoea; impotence, gynaecomastia)

Control of release of all anterior lobe hormones is exclusively humoral via 6 **hypothalamic neurohormones** (table below)

ACTH: adrenocorticotrophic hormone (corticotrophin); **TSH:** thyroid stimulating hormone (thyrotrophin); **FSH:** follicle stimulating hormone; **LH:** luteinising hormone (both FSH and LH are gonadotrophins); **GH:** growth hormone, also **STH:** somatotropic hormone (somatotropin).

Hypothalamic regulatory hormones

Hypothalamic releasing hormones (RH) and inhibiting hormones (IH) regulate the release of six anterior pituitary hormones

Abbreviation	Name	Target hormone
Releasing hormone		
CRH	Corticotrophin releasing hormone	ACTH
TRH	Thyrotrophin releasing hormone	TSH
LHRH	Luteinizing hormone releasing hormone	FSH, LH
GHRH	Growth hormone releasing hormone	GH
PRH	Prolactin releasing hormone	Prolactin
Inhibiting hormone		
GHIH	Growth hormone IH (somatostatin, SS)	GH
PIH	Prolactin inhibiting hormone	Prolactin

MOTOR DISORDERS OF THE CNS

Motor disorders of the central nervous system
Basal ganglia: functions

Afferents and efferents of basal ganglia
The major afferent excitatory **inflow** comes to the corpus striatum from the whole cortex (neurotransmitter: glutamate); an inhibitory pathway continues thence to the substantia nigra and pallidum (neurotransmitter: GABA). **Efferents** in part directly to brain stem, in part to thalamic motor nuclei (inhibitory: GABA), and from there to motor cortex; powerful feed-back loop between substantia nigra and striatum (dopaminergic Parkinsonism).

Role of basal ganglia in motor functions
Mainly participation in conversion of motor planning into movement pattern programming, i.e. definition of a temporospatial sequence of impulses which govern the executive motor centres; this includes definition of the parameters of movement such as strength, direction, speed and amplitude of movement.

Concomitant but separate **functional loops** (cortico–subcortical, trans-striatal, e.g. putamen, caudate) cooperate with afferents and efferents of the basal ganglia. This applies also to the performance of motor components.

Loop	Performance task – comment
Skeleto-motor	Preparation for movement and control of parameters of movement such as direction, amplitude, speed, strength. Organized somato-topically, with emphasis on mouth and face motility
Oculomotor	Control of eye movements, e.g. time control of saccades; cortical afferents from frontal eye field (area 8, additionally also area 7)
Complex 'associative'	Three loops are known at present: 1. dorsolateral – prefrontal, 2. orbito – frontal, 3. anterior – cingulate. Functions so far undetermined, probably participation in programming motor strategies for motivational and cognition-determined performances

Disease staging of Parkinsonism

(Reproduced after Hoehn, M. and Yahr, M. (1967) Parkinsonism: onset, progression, mortality. *Neurology (Minneapolis)*, **17**, 427–442.)

Stage I   Unilateral symptoms/signs with no or slight disability

Stage II Bilateral symptoms/signs, no postural disorder

Stage III Slight to moderate disability; disordered posture with instability on turning or external dislodgment. Employability partially preserved (job dependent)

Stage IV Full-blown picture with severe disability. Standing and walking preserved

Stage V Patient confined to wheel-chair or bed and dependent on help.

MEMORIX NEUROLOGY

Grading of disability in Parkinsonism

(Reproduced after Webster, D. (1968) Critical analysis of disability in Parkinson's disease. *Medical Treatment*, **5**, 257–282.)

I Bradykinesia of hands
0 = normal
1 = hint of slowing
2 = moderate, micrographia
3 = severe, obvious impairment of function

II Rigidity
0 = none
1 = slight
2 = moderate
3 = severe (even when treated)

III Posture
0 = normal
1 = head forward up to 12.5 cm
2 = head forward up to 15 cm; upper limbs flexed
3 = head forward more than 15 cm; upper limbs flexed above hip level

IV Upper limb swinging (walking)
0 = normal
1 = one arm reduced
2 = one arm immobile
3 = both arms immobile

V Gait
0 = normal
1 = stride down to 30–45 cm
2 = stride down to 15–30 cm
3 = stride < 10 cm; festination

VI Tremor
0 = none
1 = amplitude < 2.5 cm
2 = amplitude < 10 cm
3 = amplitude > 10 cm; writing and self-feeding impossible

VII Face
0 = normal
1 = slight lack of expression
2 = moderate lack of expression; mouth held open at times
3 = frozen face (mask), drooling

VIII Seborrhoea
0 = none
1 = increased
2 = greasy skin, lightly so
3 = greasy skin all over head

IX Speech
0 = normal
1 = hoarse, poor lilt
2 = hoarse, monotonous, indistinct
3 = palilalia

X Independence
0 = normal
1 = difficult but preserved
2 = partly dependent, everything slowed

Maximal score 30: most severe form of Parkinsonism

Idiopathic parkinsonism (Parkinson's disease): diagnostic criteria

(Reproduced after Poewe, W. and Oertel, W. *Jahrbuch Neurologie*, published by Biermann, Zülpich, 1993.)
- At least two of the cardinal signs: hypokinesia, rigidity, tremor, impaired postural reflexes
- Unilateral onset (with asymmetry during evolution)
- Positive response to L-dopa (apomorphine test, L-dopa test)
- Course $\geq$ 10 years.

Criteria of exclusion
- Encephalitis
- Treatment with dopamine receptor antagonists or calcium antagonists, drug abuse (MPTP)
- Concurrent features of cerebrovascular disease
- Course with prolonged remissions
- Oculogyric crises
- Vertical gaze palsies
- Kayser – Fleischer rings
- Cerebellar symptoms or signs
- Pyramidal tract signs
- Severe early dementia
- Severe early dysautonomia
- Gait apraxia
- Unilaterality >10 years
- Failure to respond to L-dopa
- Absence of progression over $\geq$5 years
- Incompatible findings in CT or MRI

Apomorphine test

(Reproduced after Hughes, A., Lees, A. and Stern, G. (1990) Apomorphine test to predict dopaminergic responsiveness in Parkinsonian syndromes. *Lancet*, **2**, 32–34; and (1991) Challenge tests to predict the dopaminergic response in untreated Parkinson's disease. *Neurology*, **41**, 1723–1725.)

Tests for dopaminergic responsiveness; apomorphine is a potent dopamine receptor (D1 and D2) agonist which allows prediction of result of L-dopa treatment. Premedication required because of gastrointestinal side-effects.

Premedication
- Domperidone tablets, 20 mg thrice daily for 2 days, or
- Ondansetron tablets, 4 mg 1 h before test, or 4 mg by slow iv injection immediately before apomorphine test.

Apomorphine test
- Apomorphine subcutaneous injections, 1.5 mg
  3.0 mg after 30 min interval
  4.5 mg

using alleviation of patient's individual defects for assessment of effect.

Alternative L-dopa test with laevodopa, 250 mg/carbidopa 25 mg

Reliability of tests: apomorphine test 67–90%
L-dopa test 80%

False negative and false positive test responses may occur.
A positive test does not confirm a diagnosis of idiopathic Parkinsonism.

Parkinsonism: causes
Aetiology of Parkinsonism

1. **Idiopathic Parkinsonism (Parkinson's disease)**
   (a) Juvenile form (onset before 40 years): akinetic-rigid, progressive
   (b) Senile form (after age of 70 years with features of dementia, rapid progression)
   (c) Tremor predominant symptom, often unilateral initially, fairly long-term prognosis
   (d) Rigid-akinetic form: usually bilateral, poor long-term prognosis

2. **Parkinsonism-plus syndromes (multisystem degenerations)**
   (a) Olivo-ponto-cerebellar degeneration (with cerebellar features)
   (b) Progressive supranuclear palsy (Steele–Richardson–Olszewski syndrome): associated vertical gaze palsy
   (c) Shy – Drager syndrome (dysautonomia): associated orthostatic hypotension
   (d) Striatonigral degeneration (with pseudobulbar features)
   (e) Parkinsonism – dementia – motor neuron disease complex (from island of Guam)

3. **Secondary Parkinsonism**
   (a) Metabolic causes
      (i) Wilson's disease (copper metabolism)
      (ii) Fahr's syndrome (calcium and phosphorus metabolism)
      (iii) Hallervorden – Spatz disease
   (b) Toxic causes
      (i) Carbon monoxide, manganese poisoning
      (ii) MPTP (meperidin) drug abuse
      (iii) Major tranquilizers, reserpine, metoclopramide, methyl dopa, flunarizine
   (c) Infectious causes
      (i) Acute meningoencephalitis
      (ii) Postencephalitic Parkinsonism
      (iii) Creutzfeldt – Jakob disease
      (iv) Neurosyphilis

4. **Syndromes resembling Parkinson's disease**
   (a) Vascular Parkinsonian syndrome
   (b) Post-traumatic Parkinsonism
   (c) 'Normal pressure' hydrocephalus
   (d) Parkinsonism produced by tumours
   (e) Tremor syndromes
   (f) Hypothyroidism

Glossary of Parkinsonism

Akinetic-rigid form
No, or very slight, tremor, good L-dopa response, often early onset

Akinetic crisis
Inability to move, speak or swallow

Cogwheeling
Tremulous resistance to passive movement

Drug holiday
Cessation of anti-Parkinsonian drugs (under inpatient observation)

Dyskinesias
Choreo-athetoid movements with L-dopa or dopaminergic drugs

Dystonias
Dystonic hyperkinesias (on L-dopa), usually focal (perioral, blepharospasm)

En bloc movements
Movement of whole body on turning head or trunk

End-of-dose akinesia
Akinesia following interval from last medication

Facial dissociation
Mobile lower, with rigid upper face

Freezing
Sudden immobility (e.g. in doorway or traffic) independent of L-dopa dose

Hyperkinesias
Sudden overshooting movements (especially with L-dopa overdose)

Mask
Rigid expressionless face

Micrographia
Diminishing size of handwriting

Oculogyric crises
Tonic fixing of gaze (usually upwards) in postencephalitic Parkinsonism

On-off phenomenon
Switch from normal or hyperkinetic mobility to akinesia

Oscillations
Variability of Parkinsonism, spontaneous diurnal, or from day-to-day, or after L-dopa

Palilalia
Repetitive utterances (usually linked to monotony and feeble phonation)

Paradoxical hyperkinesia
Sudden good mobility (with fear, stress, effort) independent of L-dopa intake

Peak-dose dyskinesia
Dyskinesia linked to interval from medication

Pill rolling
Coarse antagonistic finger tremor

Propulsion
Tendency to fall forward at sudden checks

Retropulsion
Involuntary stepping backwards

Rigidity
Tonic increase in muscle tone

Start hesitation
Variant of freezing

Tremor-dominant form
Relatively little rigidity or akinesia, very slow deterioration over years

Wearing off
v End-of-dose akinesia

Treatment of Parkinsonism

(Modified from Berlit, P. *Klinische Neurologie*, published by VCH, Weinheim, 1992.)

Type of drug (generic names)	Duration of action (hours)	Daily dose (mg)	Effect on Tremor	Rigidity	Akinesia	Autonomic symptoms	Particular indications	Side-effects Acute	Chronic
Anticholinergics Benzhexol Benztropine Orphenadrine Procyclidine Benztropine (injection)	1–8	5–15 2–6 100–300 10–30 1–2	++	+	0	+	Drug-induced Parkinsonism Parkinsonian crisis	Nausea, dry mouth, mydriasis, urinary retention, constipation, confusion, psychoses **Contraindication: Benign Prostatic Hypertrophy (BPH) glaucoma**	
Amantadine	2–8	100–200	(+)	(+)	++	(+)		Confusion, restlessness, psychoses, nausea **Contraindication: renal failure**	Insomnia
Dopa (and decarboxylase inhibitors) L-dopa + benserazide L-dopa + carbidopa	1–5	100–1000	(+)	+	++	(+)	Basic therapy	Nausea, tachycardia, arrhythmias, psychoses **Contraindication: cardiac failure**	Insomnia, dyskinesia, on-off phenomena, hallucinations
Dopaminergics Bromocriptine Lysuride Pergolide	1–6 2–3 7–16	2.5–30 1–5 1–5	(+)	+	+	(+)	On-off phenomena, Dopa-sparing effect of early use, tardive dyskinesia	Vomiting, hypotonia, Raynaud's syndrome, dyskinesia	Psychoses, insomnia
MAO-β inhibitors Selegiline Deprenyl	24–48	5–10 5–10	+	+		(+)	End-of-dose akinesia, wearing off, depressive symptoms	Hypotonia, nausea, dizziness, sweating	Confusion, dyskinesia

MOTOR DISORDERS OF THE CNS

Differential diagnosis of tremor
(Reproduced after Berlit, P. *Klinische Neurologie*, published by VCH, Weinheim, 1992.)

Tremor	Tremor at rest	Postural	Action	Localisation of tremor - Upper limbs	Localisation of tremor - Lower limbs	Localisation of tremor - Head	Frequency (Hz)	Peculiarities	Treatment
Essential	–	+++	+	+++	+	++	6–12	Alcohol eases; in 50% autosomal dominant inheritance	beta-blockers, primidone;
Parkinsonian	+++	+	+	+++	++	+	3–8	Hypokinesia, rigidity	Anticholinergics
Cerebellar	+	++	+++	+++	++	++	3–5	Possible associated nystagmus	Treat cause if possible. Isoniazid may ease
Senile	+	+++	++	+++	–	–	Irregular	Coarse	Beta-blockers
Metabolic (asterixis)	–	+++	+++	+++	–	–	Irregular	Flapping	According to cause, try phenytoin
Toxic	+	++	+++	+++	–	–	Irregular	Fine tremor	According to cause: exclusion
Orthostatic	Only when standing			+	+++	–	15	Collapses	Clonazepam, primidone

Symptomatic tremor: main causes

Endocrinopathy
- Hyperthyroidism
- Hypoglycaemia
- Phaeochromocytoma
- Hypoparathyroidism

Metabolic causes
- Wilson's disease
- Liver diseases
- Alcohol intoxication and withdrawal
- Uraemia

Toxic causes
- Mercury
- Lead
- Arsenic
- Carbon monoxide
- Manganese
- Cyanide
- Methanol
- Heroin (MPTP)

Medication side-effects
- Lithium
- Valproate
- Phenytoin (rarely)
- Neuroleptics
- Theophylline
- Corticosteroids
- Thyroxine
- Alpha-methyl-dopa
- Flunarizine, Cinnarizine
- Cyclosporin A
- Methotrexate
- Antihypertensives (with reserpine)
- Antipsychotics
- Tetrabenazine

Mechanisms of tremor production

1. Synchronization of motor unit discharges (physiological tremor)

2. Pathological disinhibition of long latency reflexes; tremor discharges of agonists stretches antagonists (idiopathic Parkinsonism)

3. Central oscillators: inferior olive, thalamus (essential tremor)

4. Synchronous lapses of innervation of postural musculature (asterixis, flapping tremor)

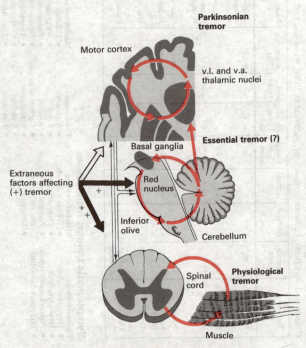

MOTOR DISORDERS OF THE CNS

Aetiology and treatment of chorea

	Aetiology	Diagnosis	Treatment
Huntington's chorea	Autosomal dominant inheritance (chromosome 4)	CT, genetic studies	Tetrabenazine, haloperidol
Sydenham's chorea	Streptococcal infections, autoimmune reaction	Laboratory tests, cardiology	Penicillin, corticosteroids
Other parainfectious choreas	Encephalitis, rubella, pertussis, diphtheria	Laboratory tests	Symptomatic
Chorea gravidarum	Pregnancy (often with history of Sydenham's chorea)	Laboratory tests	None, good spontaneous recovery, occasionally tranquillizers
Drug-induced chorea	Neuroleptics, anticonvulsants, oral contraceptives, dopaminergics, L-dopa, metoclopramide, vincristine, chloroquine, lithium	Drug history	Acute: stop drug-trigger, anticholinergics. Chronic (tardive dyskinesia): try tetrabenazine, pimozide, sulpiride
Senile chorea	Senescence	Exclude other causes	Neuroleptics (tetrabenazine)
Rare causes:			
Wilson's disease	Copper metabolism disorder	Copper, caeruloplasmin	Penicillamine
SLE	Autoimmune disease	Anti-DNA antibody studies	Corticosteroids, immunosuppressants
Thryrotoxicosis	Thyroid disease	T3, T4, TSH	Antithyroid treatment
Creutzfeldt–Jakob disease	Slow virus infection	EEG	None
Chorea-acanthocytosis syndrome	Autosomal recessive inheritance	Laboratory tests	Symptomatic
Choreoathetosis	Hereditary (paroxysmal kinesiogenic) Perinatal (anoxia, icterus neonatorum) Symptomatic (infarct, trauma, tumour)	History, examination, CT	Carbamazepine, tetrabenazine, valproate Treat cause

MEMORIX NEUROLOGY

Dystonias and dyskinesias

	Localization	Cause	Treatment
Drug-induced dyskinesias (tardive dyskinesia)	Oropharyngeal, rarely limbs	Phenothiazines, phenytoin, L-dopa dopaminergics, tricyclic antidepressants	Stop drug trigger. For acute state: anticholinergics; for chronic state: sulpiride, tetrabenazine, clozapine, valproate
Senile oral dyskinesia	Oropharyngeal	Idiopathic	Pimozide, tetrabenazine
Spasmodic torticollis	Neck muscles	Idiopathic, perinatal lesion	Haloperidol, lysuride, botulinum toxin injections, bio-feedback, benzhexol
Meige syndrome (bilateral facial spasm)	Oromandibular + eye closure	Idiopathic, in Parkinsonism	Tetrabenazine, lysuride, baclofen, lithium
Blepharospasm	Eye closure	Idiopathic, in Parkinsonism, psychogenic	Botulinum toxin injections, clonazepam, benzhexol
Hemiballismus	Unilateral arm (and lower limb)	Subthalamic infarct, bleed	Tetrabenazine, haloperidol
Athetosis	Hands and feet, uni or bilateral	Perinatal brain lesion, striatal infarction, familial, Wilson's disease	Tetrabenazine, haloperidol
Paroxysmal choreo-athetosis	Arms, legs, often triggered by alcohol	Familial, rarely sporadic	Carbamazepine, phenytoin
Chorea	Oral, limbs	Hereditary (Huntington's chorea), streptococcal infection (Sydenham's chorea), pregnancy	Haloperidol, tetrabenazine, chlorpromazine, sulpiride, penicillin (Sydenham's), benzodiazepines in pregacy
Torsion dystonia	Trunk and limbs	Idiopathic, perinatal brain damage, Wilson's disease, encephalitis	Tetrabenazine, L-dopa, bio-feedback, benzhexol
Wilson's disease	Limbs, face	Inherited copper metabolism defect	d-Penicillamine, dimercaprol, zinc sulphate
Gilles de la Tourette syndrome	Generalized, coprolalia	Idiopathic	Pimozide, haloperidol, clonidine

MOTOR DISORDERS OF THE CNS

The myoclonias
(Reproduced after Marsden, C.D. and Fahn, S. *Movement Disorders*, published by Butterworth, London, 1987.)

1. Physiological myoclonus
   Hypnagogic/waking-up myoclonus
   Startle myoclonus
   Myoclonus after muscular exertion
   Hiccough

2. Essential myoclonus
   Familial myoclonus
   Benign myoclonus
   Nocturnal myoclonus
   Hyperexplexia

3. Epileptic myoclonus
   Neonatal fits
   Myoclonic drop attacks
   Pyknolepsy
   Impulsive petit mal
   Epilepsia partialis continua
   Reflex epilepsy (photosensitive)
   Matutinal myoclonus in idiopathic epilepsy
   Progressive myoclonic epilepsy

4. Myoclonus as a feature of various underlying diseases
   Lipidoses (Tay–Sachs, etc.)
   Leucodystrophies
   Tuberous sclerosis
   Systemic atrophies (Friedreich, Pierre Marie)
   Generalized paresis of insane (syphilis)
   Whipple's disease
   Extrapyramidal syndromes (chorea, torsion dystonia, progressive supranuclear palsy, Wilson's disease)
   Malaria

5. Symptomatic myoclonus

   (a) In storage disorders
       Progressive myoclonic epilepsy (with Lafora inclusion bodies)
       Ceroid lipofuscinosis
       Sialidosis

   (b) Degenerative (hereditary)
       Dyssynergia cerebellaris myoclonica of Ramsay Hunt
       Progressive myoclonic epilepsy of Unverricht and Lundborg

   (c) Viral
       Encephalitis (lethargica, herpes simplex)
       SSPE, Creutzfeldt–Jakob disease (slow virus)

   (d) Paraneoplastic
       Myoclonus-opsoclonus syndrome (with neuroblastoma, bronchial carcinoma)

   (e) Metabolic
       Liver diseases
       Renal diseases (? dialysis)
       Hyponatraemia
       Hypoglycaemia
       Anacidotic hyperglycaemia

   (f) Toxic
       Drugs (L-dopa, bromocriptine, tricyclic antidepressants, INH, phenytoin, diclofenac, piperazine, prostaglandin)
       Convulsive poisons (strychnine, bemegride)
       Intoxications (methyl bromide, lead, mercury)

   (g) Diffuse or focal brain damage
       Hypoxia
       Trauma
       Hyperthermia
       Electric shock
       Decompression (caisson) disease
       Tumour (arteriovenous malformation)
       Thalamotomy

Myoclonia: selective treatment

	Treatment
1. Physiological myoclonus	
Nocturnal (hypnagogic and awakening) myoclonus Fright myoclonus Myoclonus after muscular exertion	No treatment required
Hiccough	Metoclopramide, carbamazepine, chlorpromazine
2. Essential myoclonus	
Familial or sporadic (5–20 years of age) Nocturnal leg myoclonus (with insomnia) Hyperexplexia (startle falls)	Clonazepam, baclofen, valproate valproate, clonazepam diazepam, phenobarbitone, piracetam
3. Epileptic myoclonus	
Infantile and juvenile epilepsies Epilepsia partialis continua Reflex epilepsies (photogenic) Progressive myoclonic epilepsy of Unverricht and Lundborg	ACTH, clonazepam, valproate Phenytoin, carbamazepine Phenytoin, carbamazepine Clonazepam, phenobarbitone
4. Reticular reflex myoclonus	
Dyssynergia cerebellaris myoclonica (Ramsay Hunt syndrome) Postanoxic reflex myoclonia (Lance, Adams) Metabolic myoclonias (uraemia, liver failure) Toxic encephalopathies (imipramine, mercury, bismuth)	Clonazepam, valproate Clonazepam, valproate Clonazepam Clonazepam
5. Symptomatic myoclonus	
Myoclonus-opsoclonus syndrome (parainfectious or paraneoplastic)	ACTH, clonazepam, phenobarbitone, propanolol
Palatal myoclonus (in brain stem infarction) Spinal myoclonus (with myelitis, spinal tumours)	Clonazepam, carbamazepine Clonazepam, tetrabenazine

MOTOR DISORDERS OF THE CNS

Cerebellar degenerations

	Aetiology and prevalence	Clinical features	Course	Treatment
Olivo–ponto–cerebellar degeneration	Autosomal dominant inheritance or sporadic	Gait and trunk ataxia, Parkinsonism, dementia	Death after 4–5 years	L-dopa, 5-hydroxy-tryptophane
Hereditary cerebellar ataxia (Nonne and Marie)	Autosomal dominant inheritance (chromosome 6)	Gait and trunk ataxia, dysarthria, spasticity, cranial nerve symptoms, dementia	Slow progression over years	5-hydroxy-tryptophane, isoniazid, clomipramine
Friedreich's ataxia	Autosomal recessive inheritance (chromosome 9)	Trunk and limb ataxia, neuropathic symptoms spasticity, scoliosis	Wheel-chair dependent before aged 30	5-hydro-xytryptophane, clomipramine, isoniazid
Late cerebellar atrophy (Marie, Foix, Alajouanine)	Mostly sporadic	Trunk, stance and gait ataxia	Normal life expectancy	5-hydroxy-tryptophane
Refsum's disease	Autosomal recessive inheritance, phytanic acid metabolic disorder	Limb ataxia, nystagmus, polyneuropathy, retinitis pigmentosa	Slow progression, treatable	Low phytanic acid diet, Vitamins A, C, E supplements; acutely: plasmapheresis
A-beta-lipoproteinaemia (Bassen-Kornzweig disease)	Autosomal recessive inheritance, lipid metabolic disorder	Limb ataxia, areflexia, polyneuropathy, skeletal deformities	Slow progression, treatable	Vitamins E, A, K supplements, low long chain fatty acid diet
Idiopathic paroxysmal ataxia	Autosomal dominant inheritance	Attacks of ataxia, dysarthria, nystagmus	Good prognosis	Acetazolamide
Dyssynergia cerebellaris myoclonica (Ramsay Hunt)	Autosomal recessive or dominant inheritance	Epilepsy, action myoclonus, ataxia, dementia	Slowly progressive	5-hydro-xytryptophane, valproate, clonazepam
Ataxia telangiectasia (Louis Bar)	Autosomal recessive inheritance (chromosome 11)	Ataxia, choreoathetosis IgA deficiency	Wheel-chair-bound in childhood	Infection prophylaxis
Shy–Drager syndrome	Autosomal recessive or sporadic	Genitourinary disorders, orthostatic hypotension, ataxia, Parkinsonism	Progressive over years	Fludrocortisone, noradrenaline, norepinephrine

Spinocerebellar disorders: genetics of biochemical abnormalities

(Reproduced after Rosenberg, R. (1991) Biochemical genetics of neurological disease. *New England Journal of Medicine*, 305, 1181–1193.)

Designation	Biochemical disorder	Age (years)	Clinical features
Lipid disorders: autosomal recessive inheritance			
Refsum's disease	Phytanic acid storage with alpha oxidase defect	10–30	Ataxia, polyneuropathy, deafness, retinitis pigmentosa, cardiac arrhythmia
Bassen–Kornzweig syndrome	Abetalipoproteinaemia	5–10	Ataxia, acanthocytosis, polyneuropathy, retinitis pigmentosa
Metachromatic leucodystrophy	Arylsulphatase A deficiency	5–20	Ataxia, polyneuropathy, spasticity, dementia
Spinocerebellar degeneration	Hexosaminidase deficiency	5–20	Ataxia, dysarthria, tremor, hyperkinesia
Adrenoleucodystrophy (X-linked recessive)	Long chain fatty acid storage	5–20	Cortical blindness, spasticity, ataxia, polyneuropathy, skin pigmentation
Carbohydrate disorders: autosomal recessive and/or mitochondrial inheritance			
Subacute necrotizing encephalopathy (Leigh)	Pyruvate carboxylase or pyruvate dehydrogenase defect	0–5	Ataxia, mental retardation, ophthalmoplegia, spasticity, optic atrophy
Eriedreich's ataxia	Lipo-amide dehydrogenase defect (in some cases)	5–15	Ataxia, dysarthria, spasticity, polyneuropathy, skeletal deformities
Kearns–Sayre syndrome	Oxidative metabolism disorder, raised serum lactate and pyruvate	20–50	Ataxia, neuromyopathy with ragged red fibres, ophthalmoplegia, retinitis pigmentosa, cardiomyopathy
Amino acid metabolism disorders: autosomal recessive inheritance			
Maple syrup urine disease	Ketoacid decarboxylase defect	5–10	Ataxia, mental retardation, epilepsy
Ataxia with reduced glutathion synthesis	Gamma-glutamyl-cysteine-synthetase defect	10–20	Ataxia, areflexia, haemolytic anaemia, psychosis
Hartnup disease	Disordered tryptophan absorption	5–25	Intermittent ataxia, spasticity, mental retardation, choreoathetosis
Olivoponto-cerebellar atrophy	Glutamate dehydrogenase defect	20–40	Ataxia, spasticity, extrapyramidal features
Disorder of immunological function: autosomal recessive inheritance			
Ataxia-telangiectasia (Louis Bar)	IgA, IgG and IgM deficiency Lymphopenia	5–12	Ataxia, areflexia, extensor plantars, telangiectasia (face and sclera)

MOTOR DISORDERS OF THE CNS

Causes of acquired cerebellar defects

1. **Toxic causes**

   Anticonvulsants (phenytoin, carbamazepine, bromide)
   Cytostatics (cytosine arabinoside, 5-fluorouracil, cisplatinum)
   Lithium, nitrofurantoin, nitrazepam, isoniazid
   Metal intoxications (lead, mercury, thallium), solvents, DDT
   Chronic alcoholism

2. **Metabolic causes**

   Deficiency of vitamin E, B_1, B_6, B_{12}
   Malabsorption, bowel disease (coeliac disease, sprue)
   Wilson's disease (copper metabolism)
   Hypothyroidism
   Mitochondrial disease
   Lipidoses

3. **Infectious causes**

   Viral encephalitis (herpes viruses, Coxsackie, ECHO, HIV)
   Creutzfeldt–Jakob disease (slow virus infection), kuru
   Cryptococcosis, toxoplasmosis
   Leptospirosis
   Tuberculosis
   Parainfectious (especially in children)
   Miller-Fisher syndrome
   Multiple sclerosis

4. **Tumour-related (paraneoplastic) causation**

   With small cell bronchial carcinoma, ovarian carcinoma, malignant lymphoma
   In children:
   Myoclonus-opsoclonus with neuroblastoma (Kinsbourne)
   Waldenström's macroglobulinaemia

MEMORIX NEUROLOGY

Differential diagnosis of dementia

	Age of onset (years)	Clinical features	Diagnostic pointers
Alzheimer type (senile) dementia	>50 (>65)	Intellectual decline, especially memory, perseveration, good façade	Temporoparietal atrophy on CT
Vascular dementia	>60	Stuttering and fluctuating course, emotional lability, poor short-term memory, nocturnal confusion, focal neurological signs, vascular factors (BP↑)	CT (SPECT, MRI, PET) show cerebrovascular defects
Subcortical encephalopathy (Binswanger's disease)	>50	Vascular dementia variant, often hypertensive, gait apraxia, urinary incontinence	CT, MRI show cerebellar white matter changes and/or subcortical lacunar infarcts
Pick's disease	45–55	Failure of routine actions, aphasia, personality change, disinhibition, grasp reflexes, oral tendencies	CT shows frontal and temporal lobar atrophy
General paresis of insane (GPI)	>30	Expansiveness, grandiose ideas, abnormal pupils, dysarthria	CSF serology positive
AIDS-dementia complex	Mostly >20	Progressive cognitive failure, apathy, headache, incoordination, tremor	Slowing of EEG, positive HIV testing
Creutzfeldt–Jakob disease	>40	Disorded intellect and consciousness, myoclonus (pyramidal, extrapyramidal and cerebellar signs), fits, rapid progression	Periodic EEG complexes
Normal pressure hydrocephalus	Any age	Intellectual decline, gait apraxia, incontinence (often history of subarachnoid bleed, trauma)	CT shows ventricular dilatation > cortical atrophy
Frontal tumour	Any age	Often papilloedema, headache, focal neurological signs, epilepsy	CT shows tumour
Craniocerebral trauma	Any age	History of trauma, often anosmia	CT may be diagnostic
Whipple's disease	Mostly >30	Eye movement disorders, myoclonus, abdominal complaints	Small bowel biopsy
Toxic encephalopathy	Any age	Often polyneuropathy, skin and mucosal changes	Examples: solvents, alcohol, lead, psychotropic drugs
Metabolic and endocrine diseases	Variable	General medical symptoms (thyroid, parathyroid, B_{12} deficiency, carcinoid, uraemia)	Appropriate laboratory tests
Accompaniment of neurological diseases	Variable	Examples: chorea, Parkinsonism, encephalitis, SLE, myoclonic epilepsy	Dependent on underlying disease

DEMENTIA

Diagnosis of Alzheimer type dementia
Definition
Slowly progressive reduction of intellectual functions and memory over a 6-month period or more. Consecutive personality changes with loss of flexibility and lability of affect.

There is impairment of at least three of five functional categories:
- orientation
- judgement
- ability to cope in the home
- ability to cope in the community
- personal care and attention.

Absence of any disorder of conscious level, primary depression and of focal neurological features.

Prevalence
5% of all aged >65 years; 60% of all demented patients aged >60 years

Senile form: onset > age 65 years, slow progression; memory defects are the presenting symptom.

Presenile form: onset aged <65 years, more rapid progression; disorientation in space and other disorders of higher mental functions, reduced motivation (frontal, temporal and parietal lobe features)

Biochemical and structural abnormalities
Specific amyloid deposition (genetically determined);
Frontal and temporal reduction of choline acetyl-transferase;
Reduction of serotonin, increased aluminium deposition.

It is imperative to exclude treatable causes of dementia.

Diagnostic procedures of exclusion	Exclude
CT, MRI	Tumour
	Hydrocephalus
	Infarction
	Haematoma
EEG	Encephalitis, epilepsy, Creutzfeldt–Jakob disease
CSF	Encephalitis, chronic meningitis, syphilis
T3, T4, TSH	Dysthyroid diseases
Vitamins B_1, B_6, B_{12}, C, folate	Wernicke–Korsakov syndrome, B_{12} deficiency
ESR, plasma electrophoresis, serology	Systemic lupus erythematosus (SLE)
TPHA, etc.	Syphilis
HIV	AIDS
Electrolytes	Hyponatraemia
	Hyperparathyroidism
Liver enzymes and LFTs	Hepatic encephalopathy
	Alcoholism
Urea, creatinine	Chronic renal failure
Glucose	Diabetes mellitus
CPK, LDH	Myoencephalopathies
Lactate, lipid electrophoresis	Mitochondrial encephalopathy
Occupational and drug history	Toxic causes

Diagnosis of vascular dementia

(Reproduced after Roman, G. *et al.* (1993) Vascular dementia – diagnostic criteria. *Neurology*, **43**, 250.)

Definition
Deterioration in memory and in intellectual abilities that causes impaired functioning in daily living; loss of memory and deficits in at least two other domains:

- orientation
- attention
- speech and language
- spatial abilities
- neuropraxis
- abstraction
- judgment
- motor control.

In addition: cerebrovascular disease (history, clinical features)
In addition: time sequence (3 months)

- Presence of all three criteria: diagnosis probable
- Presence of two criteria: diagnosis possible
- Definite diagnosis only after histological confirmation.

Criteria of exclusion
Delirium, disorders of consciousness, psychoses, severe speech disorders or other factors which preclude intellectual testing.
Presence of alternative causes of a syndrome of dementia.

Ischaemia index

(Reproduced after Hachinski, V., Iliff, L.D. and Zihlka, E. (1975) cerebral blood flow in dementia. *Archives of Neurology*, **32**, 632.)

		Points
History	Sudden onset	2
	'Stuttering' deterioration	1
	Fluctuating course	2
	Nocturnal confusion	1
	Known hypertension	1
	Past history of cerebral infarction	2
	Report of focal neurological symptoms	2
Point score >7 favours vascular dementia Point score <4 favours Alzheimer type dementia Point score between 4 and 7 borderline, overlapping, mixed form.		

DEMENTIA

Differential diagnosis of cortical and subcortical dementia
(Reproduced after Cummings (1986) Subcortical dementia. *Brittish Journal of Psychiatry*, **149**, 682.)

Criteria	Cortical dementia	Subcortical dementia
Neuropsychological criteria		
Rate of expression	Severely affected early on	Mild to moderate for long
Speed of thinking	Normal	Slowed
Memory:		
Short-term	Defect of engram formation	Clues may improve
Long-term	Gradient over time	No gradient
Speech	Naming defect, paraphasia, perceptive defect	Normal or slight, nominal defect
Visuospatial ability	Defective	Defective
Thinking	Disturbed at first, untestable later	Impaired abstraction and ability to categorize
Neuropsychiatric criteria		
Personality	Equanimity, occasional disinhibition	Apathy, irritability
Depression	Rarely	Frequently
Mania	Never	Rarely
Psychotic phenomena	Frequent: simple confusions	Common in some, with complex confusions
Motor system		
Speech	No disturbance	Dysarthria
Body posture	Remains normal for long time	Stooped or straight
Gait	Remains normal for long time	Hypokinetic or hyperkinetic
Speed of movement	Remains normal for long time	Slowed up
Abnormal movements	None, or myoclonus	Tremor, chorea, dystonia
Muscle tone	Normal at first, possibly late rigidity, 'Gegenhalten'	Abnormal: hypotonic if choreic, rigid if Parkinsonian
Localization of neuropathology	Maximal affliction of association cortex in all lobes plus hippocampus	Changes maximal in striatum and thalamus
Neurochemical defects	Alzheimer's disease: CAT ≥ AChE > somatostatin ≥ noradrenaline ≈ dopamine ≈ serotonin	Huntington's disease: GABA > angiotensin converting enzyme ≈ substance P ≈ CCK ≈ CAT Parkinsonism: dopamine ≫ noradrenaline ≈ serotonin ≈ CAT ≈ GABA ≈ CCK, metencephalin, neurotensin, bombesin Steele–Richardson syndrome: dopamine > CAT

CAT: choline acetyl-transferase; AChE: acetyl cholinesterase; CCK: cholecystokinin; GABA: gamma aminobutyric acid

Differential diagnosis of confusional states

(Reproduced after Lipowski, Z.J. (1989) Delirium in the elderly patient. *New England Journal of Medicine*, **320**, 580).

	Delirium	Dementia	Psychosis	Encephalitis
Onset	Sudden	Gradual	Sudden	Subacute
Course over 24 h	Fluctuating, often worse at night	Uniform, occasionally worse at night	Uniform	Gradually worsening
Hallucinations	Visual	None	Auditory	Rare
Illusional misconceptions	Frequent, suggestible	Rare	Systematic	Rare
Consciousness	Impaired	Normal	Normal	Often badly impaired
Attention	Badly impaired	Mostly normal	Variable	Badly impaired
Cognition	Totally impaired	Totally impaired	Selective	Totally impaired
Psychomotor activity	Variable, up or down	Mostly normal	Variable	Mostly down
Speech	Incoherent, variable rate of flow	Word finding difficulty, perseveration	Normal, rarely neologisms	Often dysphasic
Involuntary movements	Postural tremor, asterixis	None	None	None
Epileptic fits	Occasionally before onset	None	None	Frequent
Focal neurological signs	Incoordination	Rarely	None	Mostly
Fever	Rarely	None	Rarely	Often

Fits and other attacks

International classification of epileptic attacks

(Reproduced after International League against Epilepsy (1981) *Epilepsia*, **22**, 489–501.)

1. **Partial seizures or seizures beginning focally**
   (a) Simple partial seizures without impairment of consciousness
      (i) With motor symptoms (e.g. Jacksonian attacks with Jacksonian march, adversive seizures, epilepsia partialis continua, phonatory attacks)
      (ii) Sensory or somatosensory attacks (e.g. Jacksonian sensory march) or sensory symptoms (e.g. visual, auditory, olfactory or gustatory hallucinations)
      (iii) With autonomic symptoms (pallor, nausea, sweating)
      (iv) Compound forms with elementary and/or complex symptoms (amnesic, cognitive or affective symptoms, e.g. déjà-vu experience, dreamy states, fear)
   (b) Partial seizures with complex symptoms and disordered consciousness (psychomotor fits)
      (i) Simple focal attacks with subsequent disorder of consciousness
      (ii) Attacks with initial disorder of consciousness with cognitive symptoms (amnestic dreamy states, often with automatism)
      (iii) Partial seizures, secondarily generalized (e.g. grand mal with focal onset).

2. **Generalized attacks (convulsive or non-convulsive)**
   (a) (i) Absences (simple)
      (ii) Complex absences (with clonic, atonic, tonic features, automatism or incontinence)
   (b) Myoclonic attacks (includes impulsive petit mal)
   (c) Bilateral epilepsy – massive myoclonus
   (d) Tonic seizures
   (e) Tonic-clonic seizures (grand mal)
   (f) Atonic attacks (including myoclonic-atonic attacks).

3. **Unclassifiable attacks (because of inadequate information, or unclassifiability of infantile seizures)**

   Status epilepticus = repetitive epileptic attacks without complete recovery in between attacks
   (i) Generalized: absence (petit mal) status, grand mal status epilepticus
   (ii) Focal: Jacksonian status, epilepsia partialis continua.

Classification of age-related and non-age-related epilepsies and epileptic syndromes

(Reproduced after International League against Epilepsy (1985) *Epilepsia*, **26**, 268–278.)

1. **Partial seizures and syndromes**

    (a) Idiopathic with age related onset
     (i) Benign childhood epilepsy with centrotemporal spikes (Rolandic seizures)
     (ii) Childhood epilepsy with occipital spikes (Gastaut's seizures)

    (b) Symptomatic fits (depending on aetiology, clinical state and localization).

2. **Generalized seizures**

    (a) Idiopathic with age related onset
     (i) Benign familial seizures of neonates
     (ii) Benign seizures of neonates
     (iii) Benign myoclonic epilepsy of childhood
     (iv) Epilepsy with absent seizures (absence fits of childhood)
     (v) Juvenile absence epilepsy (absent seizures)
     (vi) Impulsive petit mal epilepsy (juvenile myoclonic epilepsy)
     (vii) Waking up (hypnopomic) grand mal fits
     (viii) Others

    (b) Idiopathic and/or symptomatic age related fits
     (i) Infantile spasms (West's syndrome)
     (ii) Lennox–Gastaut syndrome
     (iii) Myoclonic atonic attacks
     (iv) Myoclonic absences

    (c) Symptomatic epilepsy
     (i) Unspecified aetiology (myoclonic encephalopathy of early onset)
     (ii) Specific syndromes (vascular malformations, metabolic disorders).

3. **Fits which cannot be classified**

    (a) Generalized as well as focal
     (i) Fits of neonates
     (ii) Severe myoclonic epilepsy of childhood
     (iii) Sleep fits with spike and wave discharges
     (iv) Syndrome of aphasic fits (Landau–Kleffner)

    (b) Unsuitable for classification as either focal or generalized (e.g. grand mal in sleep)

4. **Special syndromes**

    (a) Occasional fits (febrile convulsions, alcohol withdrawal, sleep deprivation)
    (b) Oligoepilepsy (isolated and seemingly unprovoked attacks)
    (c) Reflex epilepsies with specific triggers (e.g. reading epilepsy)
    (d) Chronic progressive epilepsia partialis continua of childhood.

FITS AND OTHER ATTACKS

Common causes of fits in different age groups

In childhood
- Febrile convulsions (simple or complex)
- CNS infections
- Consequence of neonatal brain damage
- Idiopathic epilepsy
- Congenital metabolic diseases
- Neurocutaneous malformations (phakomatoses)
- Trauma.

Aged 10–25 years
- Idiopathic epilepsy
- Consequence of early brain damage
- Trauma

- CNS infections
- Vascular malformations.

Aged 25–60 years (late onset epilepsy)
- Brain tumours
- Trauma
- Inflammations (encephalitis, vasculitis)
- Consequence of earlier brain damage
- Chronic alcohol or drug abuse (occasional fits).

Aged 60+ years
- Cerebrovascular disease
- Cerebral metastases.

Acute treatment of epileptic fits

A **single grand mal** does not require specific treatment.

1. **Serial grand mal fits**
   (a) Intravenous injection of 100 ml 20% glucose solution
   (b) Rectal diazepam
   (c) If required, intravenous phenytoin 15 mg/kg, chlormethiazole or diazepam (watch respiration).
   In case of alcohol withdrawal fits:
   Vitamin B_1 100 mg iv
   Chlormethiazole: may require intensive care unit monitoring, etc.

2. **Status epilepticus (grand mal fits)**
   (a) Vitamin B_1 100 mg iv if suspicion of alcoholism
   (b) Intravenous infusion of 20% glucose plus rectal diazepam
   (c) Phenytoin 15 mg/kg injected slowly i.v. (50 mg/min) followed by maintenance dosage 100 mg 6 hourly.
   If status remains uncontrolled proceed to iv injection of diazepam or chlormethiazole, but may need intensive care (respiratory depression) and, if treatment still ineffective, proceed to general anaesthesia.

3. **Epilepsia partialis continua, partial seizure status**
   Intravenous phenytoin, as above for grand mal status epilepticus.

4. **Complex partial (psychomotor) seizure status**
   Intravenous phenytoin or diazepam, as above.

5. **Petit mal status**
   Oral valproate or ethosuximide; if necessary iv clonazepam 2 mg.

Epilepsy: first aid and prognosis
Rules of first aid for major epileptic fit

(Reproduced after Epilepsy Foundation of America. *Seizure recognition and first aid*, published by Landover, 1988.)

1. Keep calm – reassure bystanders
2. Protect patient from dangerous objects (sharp things, stones, heat).
3. Place soft object under head of convulsing person (clothing, etc.).
4. Loosen clothing at neck (tie, collar) to lessen risk of choking.
5. Place patient on side to keep airway clear.
6. Do **not** introduce gag into the mouth (risk of injury).
7. Do **not** depress tongue or attempt artificial ventilation (respiration).
8. Allow patient to recover quietly without shaking or shouting.
9. Observe patient until recovery of consciousness.
10. Do not offer drinks after the attack (danger of choking).
11. After an isolated attack the attending doctor will decide if hospital referral is required; if serial attacks happen an emergency ambulance must be called.

Pointers to a good or bad prognosis of epileptic attacks

(Reproduced after Lechtenberg, R. *The Diagnosis and Treatment of Epilepsy*, Macmillan, New York, 1985.)

Favourable	Unfavourable
Onset of epilepsy aged 1–5 years	Onset of epilepsy in first year of life
Idiopathic epilepsy	Symptomatic epilepsy (tumour, inflammation, cerebrovascular lesion)
Exclusively grand mal or complex partial seizures	Complex partial seizures in combination with tonic-clonic attacks
Normal intelligence	Mental retardation
Absence of personality disorder	Definite personality disorder
Normal EEG	EEG with temporal or frontal abnormalities
Start of treatment within 1 year	Delayed start of treatment

FITS AND OTHER ATTACKS

Medication liable to lower central epileptic threshold and cause occasional fits

1. **Withdrawal of medication:** anticonvulsants, benzodiazepines, barbiturates, chlormethiazole & hypnotics.

2. **Overdosage:** anticonvulsants (phenytoin), isoniazid, aspirin, antihistamines; insulin and hypoglycaemic agents (by causing hypoglycaemia).

3. **Intravenous infusion:** aminophyllin and theophylline, penicillin, narcotic agents (initially), lignocaine, cepitazolin, naftidrofuryl oxalate, piperazine.

4. **Intrathecal injection:** antibiotics, cytostatic agents and contrast media.

5. **Drug abuse:** cocaine, heroin, LSD.

6. **In therapeutic doses:**
   Antipsychotics (chlorpromazine, prochlorperazine etc.)
   Tricyclic antidepressants
   Muscle relaxants (baclofen, dantrolene)
   Sympathomimetics (amphetamine, ephedrine)
   Corticosteroids
   Analgesic and anti-inflammatory drugs (indomethacin, penicillamine, pentazocine, pethidine, chloroquine, phenylbutazone)
   Antibiotics and chemotherapeutic drugs (chloramphenicol, penicillin, cephalosporins, nalidixic acid, metronidazole)
   Disulfiram
   Amantadine
   Anticholinergics
   Antihistaminics
   Prostaglandins
   Cyclosporin A
   Caffeine
   CNS stimulants (strychnine)
   Digitalis
   Disopyramide
   Hexachlorophane only topical preparation.

7. **Indirectly:** parenteral infusions by overhydration; insulin and oral hypoglycaemic agents by causing hypoglycaemia.

Differential diagnosis of attacks

	Epileptic attack (grand mal)	Syncope	Psychogenic attack
Prodromes	Aura	Fading of vision, giddiness, salivation, tinnitus	Variable
Occurrence	Often during sleep or on waking	Any time	Any time
Duration	3–10 minutes	10–60 seconds	Variable, often several minutes
Clinical picture	Skin cyanotic Bitten edge of tongue Often incontinent of urine Frequently postictal injury (head, limbs, spine) Obtunded and confused for minutes Complaints of muscle aches Amnesia for all of attack	Skin pallor Very rarely tongue bitten Very rare incontinence Depends on nature of fall very rarely dazed for seconds, confused hardly ever No muscle aches Partial amnesia	Normal colour, face may flush No tongue biting, rarely central bite No urinary incontinence May have disorder of consciousness or confusion, perhaps with reactivity to environmental stimuli Variable complaints No amnesia
Laboratory tests	CPK and prolactin raised	CPK and prolactin normal	CPK and prolactin normal
EEG	May show typical epileptic changes during interval between attacks	EEG may show some slowing	EEG normal

Choice of anti-epileptic drugs

(Reproduced after Chadwick, D. (1993) in *Brain's Diseases of the Nervous System*, 10th edn, (ed. Walton, J.), Oxford University Press, and Berlit, P. *Klinische Neurologie*, published by VCH, Weinheim, 1992.)

Type of epilepsy	1st line	2nd line
Generalized epilepsy (idiopathic)		
Simple absence seizures	Sodium valproate, ethosuximide	Benzodiazepines, lamotrigine
Juvenile myoclonic epilepsy	Sodium valproate	Phenobarbitone, lamotrigine
Grand mal including awakening seizures	Sodium valproate	Carbamazepine, phenytoin, lamotrigine
Generalized epilepsy (symptomatic)	Sodium valproate, benzodiazepines	Carbamazepine, phenytoin, phenobarbitone
Partial epilepsy	Carbamazepine, sodium valproate	Phenytoin, phenobarbitone, vigabatrin
Unclassified epilepsy	Sodium valproate	Lamotrigine

Status epilepticus:	**Causes** – usually symptomatic, e.g. inappropriate anticonvulsant withdrawal, alcohol, infections, metabolic disorders, cerebrovascular and other brain diseases
	treat urgently and energetically
	  rectal diazepam as first aid in infants,
	  parenteral anticonvulsants, usually by iv drip,
	    clonazepam, or
	    diazepam, or
	    chlormethiazole, or
	    phenytoin.
	  If uncontrolled or respiratory depression: intubate and ventilate under short-acting iv barbiturate anaesthesia in intensive care unit	

Dosage and pharmacology of main anticonvulsant drugs

	Average daily dose Children	Adults	Steady state after (days)	Plasma therapeutic range*	Active non-protein-bound (%)	Rate of dose build-up	Number of doses per day
Carbamazepine	400–800 mg 30 mg/kg	600–1600 mg 20 mg/kg	4–7	3–12 mg/l 13–50 µmol/l	27–40	Slow: ½ tablet every 3 days	3–4 as short half-life; 2 of Retard preparation
Clonazepam	0.25–6 mg 0.15 mg/kg	1–8 mg 0.15 mg/kg	5–7	0.025–0.075 mg/l 0.08–0.24 µmol/l	20	Slow, to find minimal effective dose	1–4
Ethosuximide	250–1500 mg 30 mg/kg	750–2000 mg 20 mg/kg	4–8	40–100 mg/l 0.08–0.24 µmol/l	90–100	Slowly: gastric symptoms. 3-day increments	3 to improve gastric tolerance
Phenobarbitone	25–150 mg 4 mg/kg	60–180 mg 3 mg/kg	14–20	10–40 mg/l 45–170 µmol/l	50–55	Slowly, 3-day increments	1 or 2 (long half-life)
Phenytoin**	50–300 mg 5–7 mg/kg	100–400 mg 5 mg/kg	5–14	5–20 mg/l 20–80 µmol/l	7–13	No need for slow build-up	1–2 (long half-life)
Primidone	125–1000 mg 20 mg/kg	500–1500 mg 15 mg/kg	14–21 (phenobarbitone) 1–2 (primidone)	Phenobarbitone 10–40 mg/l 40–170 µmol/l Primidone 4–15 mg/l 20–70 µmol/l	Phenobarbitone 50–55 Primidone 70–100	Very slow: 3–4-day increments	3–4 (primidone half-life short)
Sodium valproate	400–1800 mg 30 mg/kg	600–2000 mg 20 mg/kg	2–6	Variable and unreliable	8–30	Slowly: bowel irritability	1–3 per day
Lamotrigine	Inadvisable	50–400 mg	1	1–3 mg/l	45	After 100 mg for 2 weeks slowly up to 200–400 mg	Twice daily: other drugs shorten half-life and may indicate double dose, e.g. valproate
Vigabatrin	0.5–3 g 50–75 mg/kg	2–4 g		Unrelated	100	0.5 g increments from 2–4 g	1–2 per day

* Plasma therapeutic ranges are recommended and not absolute values, for reference in apparent ineffectiveness or toxicity
** Phenytoin levels may alter greatly with only slight dose alterations, e.g. 25 mg/day

FITS AND OTHER ATTACKS

Anticonvulsants: possible reactions, side-effects and overdosage features

	Hypersensitivity reactions[*]	Overdosage manifestations	Side-effects (*partly dose-dependent*)	Drug-specific side-effects
Carbamazepine	Rashes in 5–10% Leucopenia in 2% Others very rare	Gait ataxia, giddiness, vomiting, diplopia, nystagmus, somnolence; rarely: irritability, more fits	Osteopathy (vitamin D deficiency), extrapyramidal dyskinesia, hair loss	At treatment onset, transient lassitude, dizziness, nausea, blurred vision. Worsening of EEG and of fits. Fluid retention, hepatotoxicity
Clonazepam	Very rarely	Somnolence, hypotonia, ataxia	Often initially somnolence; ataxia, emotional instability	Increased salivary and bronchial secretions, worse tonic fits
Ethosuximide	Very rarely	Somnolence, increased irritability	Sleep disorders, psychotic symptoms, anorexia, nausea	Hiccough
Phenobarbitone	Very rarely	**Acute:** somnolence, coma, states of agitation **Chronic:** retardation, perseveration; irritability especially in children and elderly	Osteopathy (vitamin D deficiency) neonatal bleeding tendency (vitamin K deficiency) after pregnancy-use megaloblastic anaemia from folic acid deficiency	Clubbing, Dupuytren's contracture, frozen shoulder, constipation
Phenytoin	Rashes 5% Leucopenia 2% Others very rarely	Gait ataxia, vertigo, vomiting, diplopia, nystagmus, dysarthria, tremor, somnolence, rarely irritability, increased fits; cerebellar degeneration, chronic encephalopathy	Osteopathy (vitamin D deficiency), megaloblastic anaemia, neonatal bleeding tendency (vitamin K deficiency) after pregnancy-use; extrapyramidal dyskinesias	Gingival hyperplasia (50%) coarsened facial features, chloasma, hypertrichosis, hirsutism, lymphadenopathy, hyperglycaemia
Primidone	Very rarely	As for phenobarbitone	As for phenobarbitone	At treatment start (even low doses) nausea, vomiting, drowsiness
Sodium valproate	Very rarely	Tremor, somnolence	Mostly initial and transient anorexia, nausea, vomiting. Increased appetite, obesity	Clotting disorders, toxic hepatopathy (mostly first 6 months of drug), acute encephalopathy, hair loss (mostly transient); teratogenicity (spinal dysarthism)

[*] Hypersensitivity reactions occur mostly during the first 10–20 days of treatment: exanthemata, often urticarial or morbilliform; Stevens–Johnson syndrome; exfoliative dermatitis becoming bullous; fevers; lymphadenopathy (pseudolymphoma); splenomegaly. Later: leucopenia. Very uncommonly agranulocytosis, aplastic anaemia, thrombocytopenia. Most unusual: granulomatous vasculitis

Diagnosis of sudden collapse

(Reproduced after Krause, K. (1988) Diagnostik des plötzlichen Sturzes. *Münchn M. Wschr.*, **130**, 556–557)

History	Diagnosis	Examinations and tests
Mechanical cause →	Stumble from visual disorder (strange place), or from gait disorder (Parkinsonism, sensory or cerebellar ataxia, myopathy, neuropathy, paraparesis, arthropathy); if unconscious possible superadded brain trauma	Full general, CNS and ophthalmoscopic examinations
Consciousness preserved →	1. Drop attack (consider vertebro-basilar ischaemia, suclavian steal sundrome)	Doppler sonography, possibly angiography
	2. Vestibular syncope (usually conscious)	Vestibular function tests
	3. Cataplexy with narcolepsy (differentiate laughter and startle syncope)	Neurological examination, EEG
	4. Tetany	Endocrine assessment, EMG
	5. Periodic paralysis with hypo-, hyper- or normo-kalaemia	Endocrine assessment, provocative testing with insulin/glucose, or potassium
	6. 'Claudication' of cord or cauda equina	Exercise test, myelography, MRI
	7. Transient ischaemic attacks (anterior or middle cerebral artery)	Doppler sonography, angiography
	8. Idiopathic drop attacks of women (menopausal, when walking)	
Tonic-clonic convulsions →	Grand mal (?alcohol); differentiate anoxic convulsion in syncope, especially if not recumbent	Neurological examination, EEG, possibly CT (CT obligatory if late onset or uncertain aetiology)
Myoclonus →	1. Myoclonic-atonic petit mal	Epilepsy investigations, EEG
	2. Impulsive petit mal	Epilepsy investigations, EEG
	3. Dyssynergia cerebellaris myoclonica	Epilepsy investigations, EEG
Dazed states or absences →	1. Falling attacks with temporal lobe fits	Epilepsy investigations, EEG
	2. Absence seizures with atonic components, or atypical absences	Epilepsy investigations, EEG
After sudden rising from lying or sitting or prolonged standing →	1. Orthostatic vasovagal syncope (constitutionally low BP, labile vasomotor system, prolonged recumbency, after brain trauma, infections, hypotensive medications)	Full cardiovascular testing including exercise and Valsalva tests
	2. Orthostatic hypotonia with hypovolaemia, sodium deficiency, endocrine disorders (Addison's disease, hypothyroidism)	Endocrine assessment
	3. Syncope from poor sympathetic functions (diabetes, alcohol, amyloid, porphyria, paraneoplastic (polyneuropathy, Guillain–Barré polyradiculopathy, familial dysautonomia – Riley–Day, Shy–Drager syndromes)	Neurological assessment including full peripheral neurophysiology

FITS AND OTHER ATTACKS

Diagnosis of sudden collapse (Continued)

(Reproduced after Krause, K. (1988) Diagnostik desplötzlichen Sturzes. *Münchn M. Wschr.*, **130**, 556–557)

History	Diagnosis	Examinations and tests
After extreme exertion →	Vasovagal exhaustion and fatigue reaction	
After neck manipulation →	Carotid sinus syndrome	Carotid sinus palpation Asystole ≥3s and/or RR decline ≤50 mmHg
After coughing, laughter, Valsalva manouvre →	Straining-syncope (cough-, defecation syncope): differentiate cataplexy with laughter, gelastic epilepsy as temporal lobe attack	
During or after micturition →	Micturition syncope (standing to void, in older men or children at night)	
After fright or pain →	Startle or pain syncope; differentiate cataplexy	
After quick gulping cold fluids →	Deglutition syncope (often associated with glossopharyngeal neuralgia)	
After firm eye compression →	Oculovagal syncope	Trial of eye compression
Trigeminal or glossopharyngeal neuralgia →	Syncope from trigeminal or glossopharyngeal neuralgia	
Coincidence with eating →	1. Early dumping (during eating after gastrectomy) 2. Late dumping 1½–3 h after food by hypoglycaemia	
With or after true vertigo →	Vestibular syncope (usually without loss of consciousness)	ENT examination, vestibular function tests, Doppler songraph
Screaming and rages in infants →	Breath-holding anoxic attack	Pediatric neurological or psychiatric assessment
Raised intracranial pressure →	'Cerebellar' fits (brain stem compression)	Neurological assessment urgent CT scan
Heart disease and symptoms →	Cardiogenic syncope 1. Bradyarrhythmia 2. Tachyarrhythmia (possibly pheochromocytoma) 3. Failing cardiac output	Intensive cardiovascular assessment
Psychological factors ◊	Psychogenic fainting Syncope of uncertain etiology	Psychiatric assessment

Non-epileptic attacks

1. **Syncope**
   (a) Autonomically determined syncope
      (i) Vagotonia (orthostatic, reflex)
      (ii) Sympathetic failure (polyneuropathies, Parkinsonism, Riley–Day, Shy–Drager, tabes)
      (iii) Pharmacological sympathetic blocking
      (iv) Sympathetic overactivity (heart disease, pheochromocytoma)
      (v) Central autonomic dysfunction (brain stem disease or compression)
   (b) Cardiac syncope
      (i) Cardiac arrhythmias
         Bradycardia (sick sinus syndrome, A-V block, bundle block)
         Tachycardia (supraventricular, ventricular, W-P-W syndrome)
      (ii) Reduced cardiac output
         By diminished left ventricular output (aortic stenosis, shock, obstructive cardiomyopathy)
         By reduced left ventricular filling (mitral stenosis, atrial thrombus or myxoma, cardiac tamponade, hypovolaemia)
         By disordered right heart function (pulmonary hypertension, acute pulmonary embolism)
   (c) Vascular syncope
      (i) Vertebro-basilar attacks (drop attacks), subclavian steal syndrome
      (ii) Aortic arch syndromes (Takayasu's arteriopathy)
      (iii) Dissecting aneurysm (cardiac tamponade)
   (d) Other causes of syncope
      Anoxic asphyxic syncope (breath-holding in children, asthma)
      Haematogenous anoxia (anaemia, hypovolaemia).

2. **Attacks in endocrine disorders**
   (a) Hypoglycaemic shock
   (b) Tetany and hypercalcaemia
   (c) Phaeochromocytoma
   (d) Addison's disease
   (e) Hypothyroidism (myxoedema coma).

3. **Attacks in disorders of wakefulness – sleep rhythm**
   (a) Narcolepsy (cataplectic attacks, hypnagogic hallucinations)
   (b) Pickwickian syndrome
   (c) Kleine – Levin syndrome
   (d) Periodic hypersomnia
   (e) Primary alveolar hypoventilation in sleep ('Ondine's curse')
   (f) Sleep apnoea syndrome.

4. **Psychogenic attacks**
   (a) Fear-induced respiratory 'cramps' in infants
   (b) Night terrors (in children)
   (c) Hysterical attacks (at any age).

5. **Attacks in neurological diseases**
   (a) Extrapyramidal attacks: drug-induced dyskinesias
   (b) Paroxysmal choreo-athetosis
      (i) Familial form (Mount–Reback)
      (ii) Kinesiogenic variety
   (c) Painful tonic (brain stem) spasms (especially in MS)
   (d) Complicated migraine (migraine accompagnée); basilar migraine
   (e) Somnambulism (sleep walking)
   (f) Extensor spasms (in severe diffuse brain disorders and brain stem compression).

INFLAMMATORY DISEASES OF THE CNS

Inflammatory diseases of the nervous system
Diagnosis and treatment of herpes simplex encephalitis

(Reproduced after Hacke, W. and Zeumer, H. (1986) Herpes simplex encephalitis. *Dtsch Med Wschr*, **111**, 23–25.)

Symptoms
Feverish illness with headache and nausea
Impaired higher mental functions (personality change, depressed consciousness)
Focal neurological signs (dysphasia if mainly left hemisphere)
Epileptic fits.

Investigations
CSF: Pleocytosis of 400–500, mononuclear cells
Raised protein (about 1000 mg/l)
EEG: Generalized abnormalities, focal features, especially temporal
Transient epileptic discharges
Late stage: periodic complexes

CT after 4th day ⎫ from appearance of focal neurological features temporal
MRI after 2nd day ⎭ or frontobasal necrotic lesions, frequently haemorrhagic.

Treatment
Start intravenous acyclovir as soon as herpes simplex encephalitis is suspected

Clinical course, CSF changes, CT and EEG findings in herpes simplex encephalitis

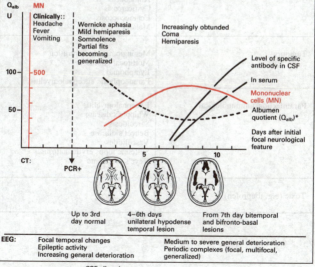

* Albumin quotient $(Q_{alb}) = \dfrac{\text{CSF albumin}}{\text{serum albumin}}$

Differential diagnosis of viral encephalitis

(Reproduced after Tyler, K. (1984) Viral encephalitis. *Seminars in Neurology*, **4**, 480–489.)

Other infectious causes	
Bacteria	Septicaemia Leptospira Tuberculosis Spirochaetes (syphilis, borrelioses) Listeriosis
Fungi	Cryptococcosis Histoplasmosis Candidiasis
Parasites	Toxoplasmosis Amoebiasis Cysticercosis Echinococcosis Malaria
Tumours	Meningiomatous infiltration Multifocal glioma Lymphoma Paraneoplastic encephalomyelitis
Parainfectious/immunological	Encephalomyelitis Whipple's disease Sarcoidosis Behçet's disease Vasculitides Systemic lupus erythematosus Reye's syndrome
Toxic (e.g. ibuprofen)	

INFLAMMATORY DISEASES OF THE CNS

Bacterial meningitis: causative organisms and treatment
(Hodges, J. and Mitchell, R. Bacterial meningitis, in *Clinical Neurology*, (eds Swash, M. and Oxbury, J., Churchill Livingstone, Edinburgh, 1991.)

	Causative organisms	Treatment
Neonates	Gram-negative enterococci, coliforms, group B streptococci *Listeria monocytogenes*	Cefotaxime + ampicillin + gentamicin
Children	*Haemophilus influenzae* *Meningococcus** *Pneumococcus* *Strepotococcus*	Cefotaxime + chloramphenicol**
Juveniles	*Meningococcus** *Pneumococcus* *Streptococcus*	Penicillin G
	Haemophilus influenzae	Triple regimen (including chloramphenicol)
Adults	*Pneumococcus* *Meningococcus** *Streptococcus*	Penicillin G
	Haemophilus influenzae	Triple regimen (including chloramphenicol)
Low resistance (alcohol, drugs, splenectomy)	*Pneumococcus* Gram-negative gut organisms *Listeria monocytogenes*	Cefotaxime + ampicillin + gentamicin**
Craniocerebral trauma/ surgery	Gram-negative gut organisms, *Staphylococcus*, *Pneumococcus*	Flucloxacillin + cefotaxime + aminoglycoside**

* Consider chemoprohylaxis for contacts with rifampicin
** Possible dexamethasone treatment under antibiotic cover

Brain abscesses: important causative organisms and antibiotics of choice

Important causes	Underlying conditions	Antibiotics/chemotherapy
Anaerobes		
Streptococci	Haematogenous, sinusitis	Cefotaxime
Bacteroides	Otitis, haematogenous	Metronidazole
Aerobes		
Proteus	Trauma, surgery	Penicillin, cefotaxime
Staphylococci	Trauma, blood-borne	Trimethoprim + rifampicin + aminoglycoside
Streptococci	Idiopathic, blood-borne	Penicillin + aminoglycoside
E. coli	Trauma, surgery	Appropriate beta-lactam + aminoglycoside
Haemophilus influenzae	Sinusitis	Cefotaxime, chloramphenicol
Mixed infections	Trauma, surgery	Cefotaxime + aminoglycoside

Entry of antibiotics into the CSF

(Reproduced after Garvey, G. (1983) Current concepts of bacterial infections of the CNS. *Neurosurgery*, **59**, 735–744.)

Good, even in absence of meningitis	Good in presence of meningitis	Moderate	None
Chloramphenicol	Penicillin	Aminoglycosides	Polymixin
Metronidazole	Ticarcillin	Clindamycin	
Cefotaxime, moxalactam	Rifampicin	Tetracycline	
Trimethoprim/sulphamethoxazole	Vancomycin		

Antibiotic treatment in neurology

	Daily dose (adults)	Dose interval for iv injection	CSF conc. (% of plasma conc.)	Mainly excreted by	Toxicity	Effective mainly against
Chloramphenicol	100 mg/kg	6 hourly	30–80	Liver	Bone marrow, allergic reactions	*H. influenzae*, *Strep. pneumoniae*, *N. meningitidis*
Benzylpenicillin	14 g	4–6 hourly	10–30	Kidneys	Allergic reactions, lowers epilepsy threshold, electrolyte disorders	Gram-positive and Gram-negative cocci, spirochaetes (treponemata)
Ampicillin	4–6 g	6 hourly	10–30	Kidneys	Allergic reactions	*Haemophilus*, *Listeria monocytogenes*
Aminoglycosides (gentamycin, tobramycin)	5 mg/kg	8 hourly	<10	Kidneys	Ototoxic, nephrotoxic, myasthenic syndrome, allergic reactions	Gram-negative organisms
Erythromycin	50 mg/kg	6 hourly	10–30	Liver	Allergic reactions, phlebitis, high tone deafness	Used in penicillin allergic reactions
Cefotaxime	6–12 g	4–6 hourly	10–20	Kidneys	Leucopenia, allergic reactions	*Haemophilus*, meningo- and pneumococcus, Gram-negative organisms, *Borrelia*
Ticarcillin	200–300 mg/kg (or 15–20 g)	4 hourly	10–30	Kidneys	As with penicillin	Gram-positive and Gram-negative organisms
Metronidazole	1.5 g	6 hourly	90–100	Liver	Gastrointestinal, leukopenia, polyneuropathy, rarely epileptic fits	Anaerobes (brain abscess)
Ceftazidime	6 g	8 hourly	10–20	Kidneys	Allergic reactions, haemolysis, nephrotoxicity	*Pseudomonas aeruginosa*

Treatment indications for neurosyphilis

(Reproduced after Prange, H. *Neurosyphilis*, VCH, Weinheim, 1987.)

1. **Absolute indications to treat**

   (a) Demonstration of *Treponema*-specific IgM antibody in serum (19S[IgM]-FTA-Abs-Test)

   (b) Finding CSF pleocytosis in presence of positive syphilis serology

   (c) When there is raised IgM in the CSF

   $$\frac{\text{IgM (CSF)}}{\text{IgM (serum)}} \times \frac{\text{Albumin (serum)}}{\text{Albumin (CSF)}} > 0.13$$

   (d) When there is increased intrathecal production of immunoglobulin G (IgGp)

   $$\text{IgGp} = \text{IgG(CSF)} - 0.43 \left[\frac{\text{Albumin (CSF)}}{\text{Albumin (serum)}} + 0.001 \right] \times \text{IgG (serum)}$$

2. **Relative indications to treat**

   (a) Demonstration of oligoclonal IgG bands in CSF with positive syphilis serology

   (b) Finding a raised index of intrathecal production of *Treponema pallidum* antibody (ITpA) >2:

   $$\text{ITpA-index} = \frac{\text{TPHA titre (CSF)} \times \text{total IgG (serum)}}{\text{TPHA titre (serum)} \times \text{total IgG (CSF)}}$$

Treatment

3×10 million IU sodium penicillin G in 100 ml of 5% glucose over 10 days

In case of allergy to penicillin:

2×100 mg doxycycline given parenterally or by mouth over 30 days

Children and pregnancy:

Erythromycin 30–50 mg/kg daily by mouth to children for 30 days;

4×500 mg daily by mouth for adults.

Neurosyphilis: diagnostic testing
(Reproduced after Roos, K.L. (1992) *Seminars in Neurology*, 12, 209.)

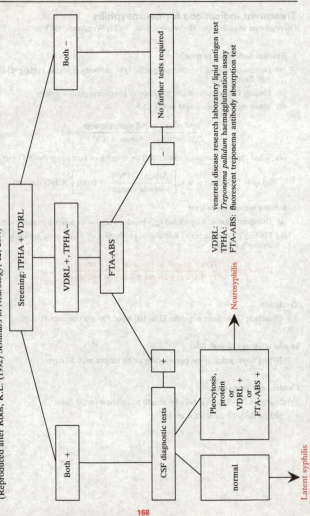

VDRL: venereal disease research laboratory lipid antigen test
TPHA: *Treponema pallidum* haemagglutination assay
FTA-ABS: fluorescent treponema antibody absorption test

INFLAMMATORY DISEASES OF THE CNS

Neurosyphilis: stages and clinical features

	Period after infection	General clinical features	Neurological features	
Primary stage	6 weeks	Primary chancre	None	
Secondary stage	6 weeks to 2 years	Rashes, lymphadenopathy, angina, condylomata	Early meningoencephalomyelitis with cranial nerve involvement (VIII, VII, III, I)	Infectious
Latent period				

Tertiary stage	5–10 years	Gummata	Meningovascular syphilis
			  Basal meningitis
			  Cerebral ischaemia
			  Meningoencephalitis
			
			Gummatous neurosyphilis
			  Cerebral
			  Spinal
				Non-infectious

Late features	10–20 years	Syphilitic aortitis
		Periostitis
		Orchitis
			Spinal syphilis (Erb's paraplegia)
			optic atrophy
			General paresis of insane (GPI)
			  Abnormal pupils (Argyll–Robertson)
			  Speech disorders
			  Personality disorders
			  Psychotic symptoms (grandiose ideas)
			
			Posterior column disorders – tabes dorsalis
			  Positive sensory features (tabetic shooting pains, (abdominal) crises)
			  Reflex changes (lost tendon jerks, exaggerated superficial abdominals)
			  Tabetic optic atrophy, abnormal pupils
			  Muscular hypotonia
			  Sensory ataxia, loss deep pain
			  Arthropathies, hyperextensibility
			  Bladder dysfunction, impotence
			  Painless perforating ulcers	

Syphilis in children: maternal transmission				
Congenital syphilis	Neonates	Pneumonia, interstitial hepatitis, osteochondritis	Rarely meningoencephalitis	
Delayed congenital syphilis	School age	Keratitis, perceptive deafness, Hutchinson's incisors, skeletal abnormalities	Juvenile tabes, optic atrophy, gummata	

Stages of HIV infection
(Reproduced from Mölling, K. *Das AIDS Virus*; published by VCH, Weinheim, 1988.)

CDC classification of HIV illness

> Stage 1: acute infection
>
> Stage 2: asymptomatic infection
>
> Stage 3: lymphadenopathy syndrome (LAS)
> persistent generalized lymphadenopathy (PGL)
>
> Stage 4: other illnesses
>
>   A Non-specific (fever for >1 month, weight loss >10%, diarrhoea >1 month)
>
>   B Neurological illnesses (dementia, myelopathy and/or peripheral neuropathy)
>
>   C Secondary infections (1. Opportunistic infections; 2. Oral leucoplakia, herpes zoster with multiple skin eruptions, recurrent *Salmonella* infections, nocardiosis, tuberculosis, oral candidiasis)
>
>   D Secondary neoplasia (Kaposi's sarcoma, Lymphoma)
>
>   E Others (lymphomata, interstitial pneumonia, illnesses resulting from failing immune responses)

Staging according to Walter Reed Hospital (WR)

WR stage	HIV test	Chronic lymph-adenopathy	T helper cells (CD4) (/mm^3)	Delayed hyper-sensitivity	Erythema	Opportunistic infections
0	−	−	>400	Normal	−	−
1	+	−	>400	Normal	−	−
2	+	+	>400	Normal	−	−
3	+	±	<400	Normal	−	−
4	+	±	<400	Partial	−	−
5	+	±	<400		Complete skin anergy and/or erythema	−
6	+	±	<400	Partial to complete	±	+

▨ Relevant parameters for staging

INFLAMMATORY DISEASES OF THE CNS

Neurological complications in AIDS

(Reproduced after Fischer, P. and Enzensberger, W. (1987) Neurological complications in AIDS. *Journal of Neurology*, **234**, 269–297.)

1. **Diseases caused by HIV** (human immunodeficiency virus)
    Acute HIV meningoencephalitis (at time of infection or seroconversion)
    AIDS-dementia complex (chronic AIDS-encephalopathy) CDC criteria
    Chronic HIV meningitis (in pre-AIDS patients)
    Vacuolar HIV myelopathy (in AIDS stage)
    HIV polyneuropathy (in AIDS stage)
    HIV myopathy.

2. **Illnesses from opportunistic infection in immunodeficient states**

Illness	Treatment
Parasitoses	
Toxoplasmosis	Pyrimethamine + sulphadiazine
Mycoses	
Cryptococcosis (*Cryptococcus neoformans*)	Amphotericin B + 5-fluoro-cytosine
Candidiasis (*Candida albicans*)	Ketoconazole (imidazole)
Aspergillosis (*Aspergillus fumigatus*)	As in cryptococcosis
Viral infections	
Cytomegalovirus (CMV)	DHPG (Foscarnet, Gancyclovir)
Herpes simplex virus (HSV)	Acyclovir
Varicella-zoster virus (VZV)	Acyclovir
Papova virus: progressive multifocal leucoencephalopathy	No known treatment
Bacterial infections	
Tuberculosis	Antitubercular bacteriostatic drugs
Listeria monocytogenes	
Treponema pallidum	
Escherichia coli	Antibiotics
Salmonella species	
Nocardia asteroides	

3. **CNS malignancies**
    Primary CNS lymphoma
    Systematic lymphoma with CNS involvement
    Kaposi sarcoma with CNS involvement (unusual)

4. **Cerebrovascular events**
    Cerebral infarction (in cases of vasculitis)
    Intracerebral haemorrhage.

Stages of AIDS – Dementia Complex (ADC)
(Reproduced after American Academy of Neurology (1989) HIV infection and the nervous system. *Neurology*, **39**, 119–122.)

ADC stage	Criteria
0	Normal mental and motor functions
0.5 (subclinical)	Minimal symptoms (concentration, cognition, personality change, motor slowing) or clinical signs (changed reflexes, primitive reflexes)
1 (mild)	Mental and/or motor limitations: no restrictions in job or activities of daily living in the absence of unusual stresses
2 (moderate)	Patient remains ambulant and capable of self-care but can no longer work
3 (severe)	Severe limitation of mental functions (dementia, mutism) or of motor functions (paraparesis, incontinence), depends on help from third persons
4 (final)	Approaching decerebrate state

Causes of chronic meningitis
(Reproduced after Wilhelm, C. and Marra, C. (1992) Chronic meningitis. *Seminars in Neurology*, **12**, 234.)

Pathogenic causation
- Tuberculosis
- Syphilis
- Mycoses
- Borreliosis
- Brucellosis
- Toxoplasmosis
- Leptospirosis
- Infective endocarditis
- Parasitoses
- HIV
- Enteroviruses
- Epstein–Barr virus

Rheumatic diseases
- SLE
- Sjögren's disease
- Mixed connective tissue disease
- Rheumatoid arthritis
- Behçet's disease
- Reiter's syndrome

Other non-infectious illnesses
- Sarcoidosis
- Vasculitides
- Neoplasia (cerebral tumours or paraneoplastic)
- Vogt–Koyanagi–Harada syndrome
- Fabry's disease (angiokeratoma corporis diffusum)
- chronic benign lymphocytic meningitis

Drug-induced
- Ibuprofen
- Azathioprine
- INH
- Trimethoprim
- Penicillin
- Sulindac

CEREBROVASCULAR DISEASES

Classification of cerebral ischaemia

By criteria of time

History, CT
TIA (transient ischaemic attack): maximal duration 24 hours
RIND (reversible ischaemic neurological deficit): maximal duration 1 week
Infarct (persistent symptoms, signs)

By criteria of localization

Examination, CT, MRI
Anterior (carotid) circulation
- anterior cerebral artery
- middle cerebral artery (posterior circulation)
posterior circulation (vertebrobasilar)
- posterior cerebral artery
- pons
- medulla
- cerebellum

By criteria of pathogenesis

CT, MRI
Microangiopathy:
Territorial infarct: embolic, thrombus
End artery infarct } haemodynamic
Borderzone infarct

Microangiopathy:
Lacunar infarcts } subcortical arteriosclerotic
White matter   } encephalopathy
dystrophy

By angiological criteria

Sonography, angiography, laboratory tests
Macroangiopathy:
Extracranial vessels
Intracranial vessels
- plaque
- stenosis
- ulceration
- collateralization
- occlusion
- dissection
- dysplasia
- arteritis

Microangiopathy with hypertension
Diabetes mellitus
Other angiopathies (collagenoses, etc.)

By cardiological criteria

ECG, echocardiography
possible cardiac cause of embolism
    endocarditis
    congenital defect
    cardiac arrhythmia
    cardiomyopathy
    mitral valve prolapse
    myocardial infarction

concurrent heart disease: coronary disease, cardiac arrythmia

Risk factors, concomitant diseases and findings which increase risk of cerebral infarction

Risk factors	Risk of cerebral infarction
Hypertension	6-fold increase, rising with age
Diabetes mellitus	3-fold increase
Smoking	3-fold increase in cigarette smokers
Hyperlipidaemia	2-fold increase, mainly aged >50 years
Oral contraceptives	2–3-fold increase
Alcohol abuse	2-fold increase (in younger persons)
Concomitant illnesses	
Myocardial ischaemia (coronary disease)	6-fold increase, rising to 10-fold if concurrent cardiac arrythmia
Thrombotic vascular disease of legs	2-fold increase
Migraine	Potentiates other risk factors (contraceptives, smoking)
Obesity	No definite effect
Findings	
History of TIA	4% per annum
Asymptomatic extracranial carotid stenosis of <70%	2% per annum
Stenosis of >80%	4–8% per annum
Ulcerated plaque	4–8% per annum
Polycythaemia	Up to 2-fold
Hyperuricaemia	No definite effect

MEMORIX NEUROLOGY

Diagnosis of cerebral infarction

History	
Description of symptoms	Was the deficit truly ischaemic?
	Differential diagnosis: hypotension, cardiac disorder, epilepsy
	Anterior or posterior circulation
Duration of symptoms	TIA, RIND, infarct
Concomitant symptoms	Headache (haemorrhage, tumour, migraine)
	Disordered consciousness (bleed, tumour, fit, basilar artery, heart disease)
	Cardiac symptoms (heart disease)
	Vertigo, nausea, vomiting (vertebro-basilar, tumour, migraine)
Onset in time	During sleep
	Provoked by exertion
Course	Increase/decrease (march of convulsion, progressive stroke)
	Recurrences (stuttering)

Clinical findings	
Neurological signs	Persistent symptoms and signs
	Anterior or posterior circulation
	Accompanying features (unconsciousness, papilloedema)
Cardiovascular signs	Neck vessels (bruits, palpability, collaterals?)
	Blood pressure (raised? right-left discrepancy?)
	Heart (disorders of rhythm, murmurs)
	Peripheral vessels (subclavian, leg arteries)

Laboratory tests	
Basic diagnostic test	Full blood count, ESR, haematocrit
	Electrolytes, creatinine, urea
	Glucose
	Clotting studies
	Cholesterol, triglycerides
	Uric acid
Additional tests	Blood clotting analyses (antithrombin III, fibrinogen anti-phospholipid antibodies)
	Vasculitis tests
	Lipid electrophoresis
	T3, T4
	Serology (syphilis, borrelioses, viruses)

Further diagnostic investigations
Doppler sonography, duplex sonography, transcranial Doppler sonography
CT, (MRI), (SPECT), (PET)
Angiography
Neurophysiology (EEG, evoked potentials, transcranial magnetic stimulation)

Diagnostic value of investigations in cerebral infarction

	CT	Doppler sonography	B mode	Angio-graphy	MRI	Other
TIA in carotid circulation	++	+++	+++	+	(+)	Cardiac investigations
TIA in posterior circulation	+	+++	++	(+)	++	4 X-ray views of cervical spine, subclavian investigations
Infarct in carotid territory	+++	+++	++	+	(+)	Cardiac investigations
Cerebellar infarct	+++	++	+	(+)	++	Re-check CT (obstructive hydrocephalus)
Brain stem infarct	+	++	++	(+)	+++	Exclude basilar stenosis
Multifocal ischaemia	+++	++	++	(+)	(+)	Cardiac investigations, exclude vasculitides

+++: obligatory investigation
++: important investigation
+: additional investigation
(+): only if specifically indicated

CEREBROVASCULAR DISEASES

Important collaterals for cerebral blood supply

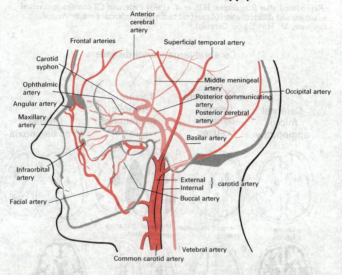

Internal to external carotid circulation
Ophthalmic artery

Anterior (carotid) to posterior (vertebro-basilar) circulation
Posterior communicating artery (siphon to posterior)
Choroidal arteries (siphon to posterior)
Occipital artery (external carotid to vertebral)
Corpus callosum anastomoses (anterior to posterior)
Leptomeningeal anastomoses (anterior to posterior, middle to posterior)

Interhemispheric
Anterior communicating artery (right anterior to left anterior)

MEMORIX NEUROLOGY

Pattern of CT changes in cerebral infarction

(Reproduced after Ringelstein, E.B. *et al.* (1985) Pattern of CT changes in cerebral infarction and differentiation of cerebral hemisphere infarcts. *Fortschr Neurol Psychiatr*, **53**, 315–336 (in German).)

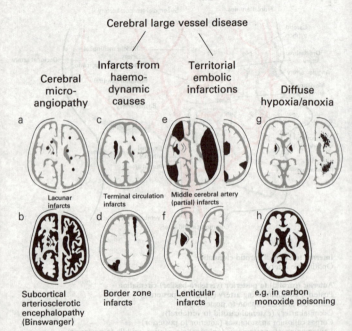

a. Subcortical lacunar infarcts
b. Subcortical arteriosclerotic encephalopathy (Binswanger's disease)
c. Subcortical terminal white matter circulation infarcts (long penetrating arteries)
d. Border zone infarcts between two arterial territories
e. Territorial infarctions from thrombotic or embolic occlusion of large intracranial arteries and branches
f. Territorial infarction in lenticulostriate artery territory (extensive lenticular infarct)
g. Cerebral atrophy and bilateral terminal circulation infarcts after anoxia
h. Bilateral symmetrical pallidal necrosis after carbon monoxide poisoning.

CEREBROVASCULAR DISEASES

Localizing value of clinical pictures

Clinical features	Localization of CVA
Monoparesis	Cortical
Sensory-motor hemiplegia 　Worse in upper limb 　Worse in lower limb	Supratentorial 　Middle cerebral artery 　Anterior cerebral artery territory
Homonymous hemianopia Diplopia, vertigo Impaired consciousness	Posterior or middle cerebral artery Vertebro-basilar territory: medulla
Paraparesis	Vertebro-basilar territory: pons
Crossed syndromes	Vertebro-basilar territory: medulla
Eye movement disorders	Mesencephalon, pons
Hemiataxia	Cerebellum (or connections)

Vascular territories in CT

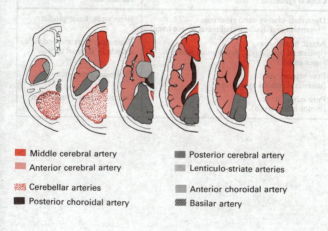

- ■ Middle cerebral artery
- ■ Anterior cerebral artery
- ▒ Cerebellar arteries
- ■ Posterior choroidal artery
- ■ Posterior cerebral artery
- ■ Lenticulo-striate arteries
- ≡ Anterior choroidal artery
- ▓ Basilar artery

Thalamic infarcts

Affected area	Blood supply	Clinical features
Posterolateral	Thalamogeniculate artery (from posterior cerebral artery)	Persistent contralateral hemianaesthesia with deep sensations impaired, spontaneous pain, fleeting contralateral hemiparesis
Anterolateral	Thalamic perforating arterioles (from posterior communicating artery)	Disorientation, reduced drive, tremor, choreo-athetoid restlessness
Dorsomedial	Posterior thalamic perforating arteries (from posterior cerebral artery or to both sides from basilar termination)	Amnesic syndrome, dementia (if bilateral infarction), vertical gaze palsy, III nerve palsy

Lacunar infarcts

Clinical syndrome	Localization
Dysarthria-clumsy hand syndrome (dysarthria and dysdiadochokinesis of one hand)	Brain stem, basal ganglia
Ataxic hemiparesis (ipsilateral hemiataxia, hemiparesis worse in lower limb)	Brain stem (cerebral peduncle included), internal capsule
Pure sensory stroke (unilateral sensory symptoms)	Thalamus, brain stem
Pure motor stroke (motor hemiparesis)	Internal capsule, brain stem

CEREBROVASCULAR DISEASES

Percentage frequency of arteriosclerotic obstructions in extracranial arteries to the brain and in the circle of Willis

(Modified from Hass, W. et al. (1968) Joint study of extracranial occlusion. *Journal of the American Medical Association*, **203**, 961.)

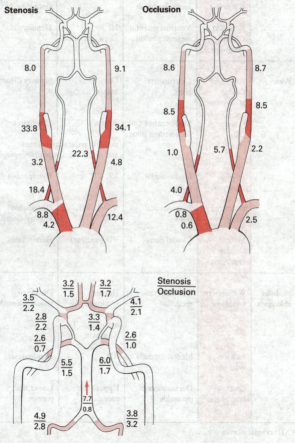

Crossed brain stem syndromes

	Eponym	Localisation	Ipsilateral	Contralateral
Midbrain	Weber's syndrome	Ventral mesencephalon	III	Hemiparesis (including face)
	Benedikt or Claude syndrome	Ventrosegmental mesencephalon	III Skew deviation	Hemiataxia
Pons	Raymond–Céstan syndrome	Laterorostral pons	Gaze palsy, ataxia	Sensory disorder
		Mediorostral and paramedian pons	Ataxia possibly palatal myoclonus and internuclear ophthalmoplegia	Hemiparesis
	Foville syndrome	Mediocaudal pons	VI, VII	Hemiparesis
	Gasperini syndrome	Laterocaudal pons	V, VI, VII, VIII	Dissociated sensory disorder
	Millard–Gubler syndrome	Caudal pons	VII (nuclear)	Hemiparesis
Medulla oblongata	Wallenberg syndrome	Dorsolateral medulla	Horner's syndrome, V (sensory), nystagmus, IX, X, ataxia	Dissociated sensory disorder
	Jackson syndrome	Medial medulla	XII	Hemiparesis
	Cruciate hemiplegia	Decussation of pyramids	Upper limb paresis	Lower limb paresis

I–XII: cranial nerves

CEREBROVASCULAR DISEASES

Vascular territories of the three main cerebral arteries

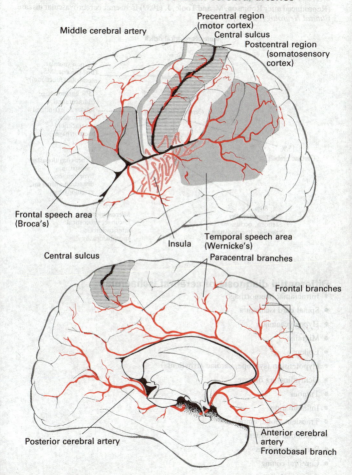

Differential diagnosis of stroke

(Reproduced after Robinson, M. and Toole, J. (1989) Ischaemic cerebrovascular disease. *Clinical Neurology*, **2**, 39.)

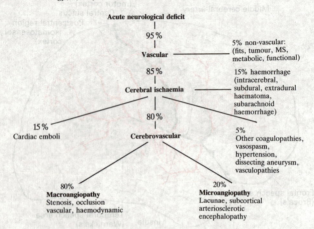

Differential diagnosis of cerebral ischaemia

- Intracranial haemorrhage
- Spinal cord ischaemia
- Hypoglycaemia
- Migraine
- Epilepsy
- Hypotension (syncope, cardiac arrhythmia)
- Demyelinating disease
- Tumour
- Inflammation
- Transient global amnesia
- Vestibular disorders
- Periodic paralysis
- Cerebral coning
- Functional disorders.

CEREBROVASCULAR DISEASES

Principles of management of cerebral infarction

Improve cerebral blood flow	Lessen tissue vulnerability
• Removal of obstruction	• Maintain normal blood glucose levels
• Improve collateral flow	• Prevent, or treat, cerebral oedema
• Improve perfusion parameters	• Hypothermia (reduce any fever)
• Maintain blood pressure (lower head)	

Anticoagulation in acute cerebral infarction

Indications

1. *Recommended on the basis of controlled trials:*
   Established atrial fibrillation
   Cardiogenic cerebral embolism (from known site in the absence of endocarditis)
   Venous sinus thrombosis.

2. *Recommended on the basis of non-blinded retrospective trials:*
   Basilar stenosis/occlusion causing acute ischaemia; possibly thrombolysis
   Other intracranial stenoses/occlusions with acute ischaemia
   Dissection of arteries supplying brain.

3. *Recommended on empirical grounds:*
   Coagulopathies
   Cerebral infarction with gross extracranial stenoses
   Progressive/labile cerebral infarction.

Preconditions
CT
Normal clotting screening tests
Exclusion of sources of internal bleeding
Absence of malignant hypertension
Age (?)

Hazards
Haemorrhagic transformation of infarct (15–50%, with clinical signs in up to 4%)
Other bleeds (risk about 5% per annum, increasing after first 6 months)
Thrombocytopenia
Platelet activation (?)

Indications for internal carotid endarterectomy

(Reproduced after Berlit, P. and Storz, W. (1989) On the indication and evaluation of internal carotid thromboendarterectomy. *Dtsch Med Wschr*, **114**, 471–474 (in German); ECST (1991) *Lancet*, **337**, 1235–1243.)

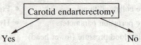

	Yes	No
Clinical symptoms	Focal neurological symptoms (sensory, motor, dysphasic, amaurosis fugax, hemianopia in internal carotid territory	Absence of focal neurological symptoms (vertigo, falls, disorders of consciousness)
Computerized tomography (CT)	Old infarct(s) in intracranial territory, infarction of terminal or border zone regions	Extensive fresh infarction, lacunar infarcts, Binswanger's disease
Ultrasound of great neck vessels, arteriography	Stenosis ≥70% and absence of relevant intracranial stenoses	Stenosis of <70% or plaque
General medical assessment	Reasonable anaesthetic and surgical risk for age	Increased complication risk of anaesthesia and surgery
Constellation of findings	Clinical symptoms and signs and arteriography concur	Disagreement of clinical and arteriographic findings

Indications for endarterectomy in internal carotid stenosis

1. Angiographic proof of severe stenosis or ulcerated plaque (arterial digital subtraction angiography) ≥70%: 30–70% debatable; no indication if <30%.

2. Transient ischaemic attacks in vascular territory distal to lesion
   or
   embolically caused infarction in appropriate territory (CT)
   or
   infarction from haemodynamic causes in appropriate territory (CT) with proof of haemodynamically relevant stenosis in Doppler sonography.

3. Additional stenoses in anterior and posterior circulations have been excluded.

4. Serious cardiac disorders have been excluded.

5. There is no CT evidence of intracerebral haemorrhage, or of extensive fresh infarction or of lacunae (microangiopathy).

6. The perioperative mortality and complication rate of the centre concerned is acceptably low (3–5%).

CEREBROVASCULAR DISEASES

Subclavian steal syndrome

Basilar artery

Right vertebral artery

Retrograde blood flow in left vertebral artery

Common carotid arteries

Innominate artery

Proximal occlusion of left subclavian artery

Aorta

Left-sided subclavian steal syndrome with blood supply to left arm from ipsilateral vertebral artery

Scale for quantification of neurological deficits in the course of infarction: NIH stroke scale

(Reproduced after Biller, E.B. *et al.* (1987) 112th Meeting of American Neurological Association, San Francisco.)

Conscious level
0 = awake
1 = drowsy, somnolent
2 = stupor
(rousable to correct localization of painful stimulus)
3 = no reaction, or extensor or flexor spastic response

Response to questions (month, age)
0 = both answers correct
1 = one answer correct
2 = both answers wrong or no response

Reaction to verbal order (open or shut eyes, hand grip)
0 = both correct
1 = one correct
2 = no reaction or incorrect action

Eye movements
0 = normal
1 = partial gaze palsy
2 = complete gaze palsy (also to oculocephalic manoeuvre)

Visual field
0 = full
1 = incomplete hemianopia
2 = complete hemianopia

Facial palsy
0 = normal
1 = slight
2 = moderate
3 = complete

Attempted posture (affected arm)
0 = unremarkable (10 s)
1 = pronation
2 = 90° posture fails <10 s, rapid droop
3 = postural attempt fails

Attempted posture (affected lower limb)
0 = unremarkable (5 s)
1 = droops
2 = lower limb flops (5 s)
3 = postural attempt impossible

Limb ataxia (affected side)
0 = normal
1 = one limb ataxic
2 = both limbs ataxic

Sensation
0 = normal
1 = hypesthesia
2 = anaesthesia

Neglect
0 = normal
1 = partial neglect (inattention) one side
2 = complete hemi-neglect (several sensory modalities)

Dysarthria
0 = normal
1 = dysarthric but easily understood
2 = severe dysarthria, barely intelligible

Aphasia
0 = normal
1 = mild dysphasia (word finding difficulty, paraphasia, grammatical errors)
2 = motor (Broca) or sensory (Wernicke) aphasia or variants
3 = complete aphasia, muteness

Scale for assessment of independence after cerebrovascular accident (Barthel scale)

(Reproduced after Barthel, D. and Mahoney, F. (1965) Functional evaluation. *State Medical Journal*, **2**, 61–64.)

Eating
10 = independent (with aids)
 5 = needs help (e.g. cutting food)
 0 = needs to be fed

Washing
 5 = possible without help
 0 = feasible only with help

Bodily care (brushing teeth, combing hair, shaving)
 5 = possible without help
 0 = feasible only with help

Dressing
10 = independent
 5 = possible only with assistance
 0 = totally dependent

Bowel control
10 = independent of aids
 5 = occasional incontinence, requires assistance
 0 = incontinent

Bladder control
10 = independent
 5 = occasional incontinence, requires assistance
 0 = incontinence or indwelling catheter

Use of toilet (lavatory)
10 = independent use of lavatory or bedpan
 5 = requires help
 0 = bed-ridden, totally dependent

Wheel-chair to bed transfer
15 = independent use of wheel-chair
10 = minimal help needed
 5 = can sit but needs much assistance
 0 = bed-ridden

Mobility
15 = can manage 50 steps (walking aids but no frame)
10 = manages 50 steps with help (accompanying person, frame)
 5 = can manage distance of 50 paces in a wheelchair
 0 = no longer able to manoeuvre wheel-chair

Climbing stairs
10 = independent with holds and walking aids
 5 = possible with help from accompanying person
 0 = impossible

MEMORIX NEUROLOGY

Anatomy of cerebral venous drainage

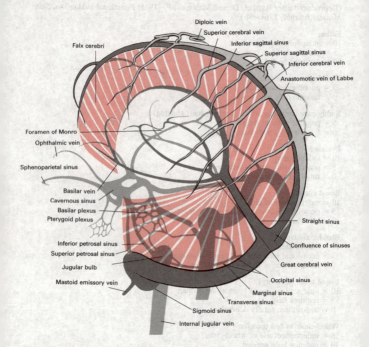

CEREBROVASCULAR DISEASES

Symptoms and signs of cerebral venous sinus thrombosis

(Reproduced from Berlit, P. *Klinische Neurologie*, published by VCH, Weinheim, 1992.)

General features
- Headache with nausea and vomiting
- Mild to marked pyrexia
- Raised ESR, leucocytosis
- Signs of raised intracranial pressure (papilloedema, disordered consciousness)
- Convulsive seizures (focal > generalized, often with postictal pareses)
- Disorientation, psychiatric symptoms.

Focal features
- Superior sagittal sinus thrombosis
  Lower limb palsy, tetraparesis, bladder dysfunction
- Transverse sinus thrombosis
  Cranial nerve deficits IX, X, XI
  Soft tissue swelling in mastoid region, possibly VI nerve palsy (inferior petrosal sinus)
- Cavernous sinus thrombosis
  Cranial nerve deficits III, IV, V, VI,
  Proptosis, lid oedema, chemosis, papilloedema
- Cortical vein thrombosis
  Alternating hemipareses, epileptic fits
- Deep cerebral veins
  Bilateral extrapyramindal features, rigidity.

Venous sinus thrombosis: causes and associated disorders

Haematological disorders and defects
- Antithrombin III deficiency
- Protein C and S deficiency
- Haemolytic anaemia
- Paroxysmal nocturnal haemoglobinuria
- Idiopathic thrombocythaemia

- Cryofibrinogenaemia
- Antiphospholipid antibody syndrome
- Disseminated intravascular coagulation
- Polycythaemia, leukaemias
- Nephrotic syndrome.

Immunological disorders
- Behçet's disease
- Wegener's granulomatosis
- Crohn's disease

- Sarcoidosis
- Paraneoplastic
- Ulcerative colitis.

Hormonal disorders and deviations
- Oral contraceptives
- Pregnancy, postpartum state (puerperium)

- Androgen therapy.

Infections
- Meningitis
- Otitis media, mastoiditis

- Aspergillosis
- Trichinosis

Others
- Lymphoma, leukaemia
- Local tumour invasion (carcinomatosis)
- Arteriovenous malformation
- Craniocerebral trauma

- Budd – Chiari syndrome
- Cachexia, marasmus, dehydration
- Cardiac/pulmonary diseases.

Subarachnoid haemorrhage

Grading of subarachnoid haemorrhage
(Reproduced after Hunt, W. E. and Hess, R. M. (1968) Surgical risk as related to time of intervention in the repair of intracranial aneurysm. *Journal of Neurosurgery*, **28**, 14.)

Grade 1: minimal headache, mild meningismus

Grade 2: severe headache, neck rigidity, cranial nerve palsies but no other neurological deficit

Grade 3: drowsy, confused, or mild focal deficit

Grade 4: stupor, moderate to severe pareses, early decerebrate rigidity, autonomic disturbances

Grade 5: deep coma, decerebrate rigidity.

Preconditions for early surgery after subarachnoid haemorrhage

Establishment of diagnosis and surgery within 72 h of headache onset

Angiographic demonstration of aneurysm

Patient graded 1–3 by Hunt and Hess scale.

Preconditions for late surgery after subarachnoid haemorrhage

Bleed at least 14 days earlier

Angiographic demonstration of aneurysm

Exclusion of vascular spasms by transcranial Doppler sonography

Actual clinical grade 1–3 by Hunt and Hess scale regardless of initial score.

CEREBROVASCULAR DISEASES

Common sites of cerebral aneurysms

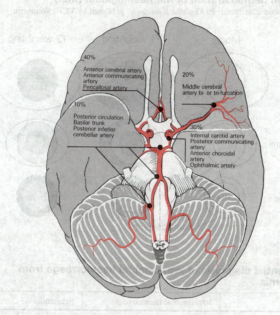

Neurological defects from cerebral aneurysms

Site of aneurysm	Symptoms and signs
Posterior communicating artery	Painful III nerve palsy, usually with dilated pupil
Internal carotid artery supraclinoid portion	Visual field defects or optic atrophy (compression of optic nerve or tract or chiasm), occasionally VI nerve palsy
infraclinoid portion	Paresis of III, IV and/or VI nerves, disturbed sensation and pain in first two trigeminal divisions
Anterior communicating artery	Bitemporal hemianopia and other visual field defects
Basilar artery	VI nerve palsy, rarely also CNS motor deficits

Estimation of age of intracerebral haemorrhage by MRI through demonstration of methaemoglobin (met)

(Reproduced after Berlit, P. *Klinische Neurologie*, published by VCH, Weinheim, 1992.)

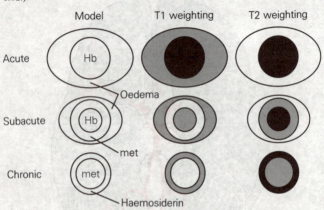

Differential diagnosis of intracerebral haemorrhage from ischaemia

	Intracerebral haemorrhage	Ischaemia
Onset	Over minutes to hours, progressive	Abrupt
TIA	None	Possibly
Headache/vomiting	Frequently	Rarely

CEREBROVASCULAR DISEASES

Intracerebral haemorrhage: frequency and causes in various sites

(Reproduced after Schütz, H. *Spontane Intrazerebrale Haematome*, published by Springer, Berlin, 1988.)

		Frequency (%)	Causes
Basal ganglia		60	Hypertension (70%), tumour (3%), aneurysm (2%), angioma (1%), (AVM) (1%)
	Total	10	
	Putamen	25	
	Thalamus	20	
	Other	5	
Lobes of cerebrum		30	Hypertension (35%), angioma (15%), aneurysm (10%), tumour (5%)
	Frontal	8	
	Temporal	12	
	Parietal	5	
	Occipital	5	
Infratentorial		10	Hypertension (70%), angioma (20%)
	Cerebellum	5	
	Pons	5	
Total		100	Hypertension 60%, aneurysm 20%, angioma 10%, tumours 5% (melanoma and bronchial, metastases, glioblastoma), anticoagulants 5%, haemorrhagic diatheses 5%, other (vasculitis, amyloid, angiopathy)

Spontaneous intracranial bleeding: diagnostic procedures

Computerized tomography	Laboratory tests	Clinical history
Localization	Clotting	Hypertension
Ventricles and subarachnoid space	Inflammation	Alcohol
Brain substance, before and after contrast	Liver functions	Coronary artery disease
Re-check for progression, if indicated also MRI	Aldosterone VMA	Medicaments, drugs (anticoagulants in particular)

Occasionally cerebral angiography may be indicated or rectal biopsy (? amyloidosis)

Main clinical features of intracranial haemorrhage

(Reproduced after Schültz, H. *Spontane Intrazerebrale Haematome*, published by Springer, Berlin, 1988.)

	Focal neurological symptoms and signs	Additional features	Epileptic attacks	Mortality (approximate %)	Severe residual disability (approximate %)
Basal ganglia haemorrhage					
Putamen	Variable hemiparesis and dysphasia	Conjugate eye deviation, often disordered consciousness	Rarely	40–50	50
Thalamus	Variable hemiparesis, vertical gaze palsy, myosis	Possibly later thalamic syndrome	–	5	40
Head of caudate nucleus	Organic personality disorder with disorientation, possibly hemiparesis	Headache, meningismus	–	–	20
Lobar haemorrhage					
Frontal	Motor hemiparesis worst in UL	Possibly reduced consciousness	Rarely	30	40
Temporal	Brachiofacial hemiparesis	Rare, reduced consciousness	Often	40	30
Parietal	Mainly sensory hemisyndrome		Often	30	20
Occipital	Homonymous hemianopia		–	20	10
Infratentorial					
Cerebellum	Gait, trunk and possibly also limb ataxia	Headache, vomiting, vertigo, dysarthria	–	20	20
Pons Paramedian	Horizontal gaze palsy, ocular bobbing, 1½-syndrome, pinpoint pupils, tetraparesis	Mostly reduced consciousness, occasionally hyperthermia, respiratory disorder, gastrointestinal bleeding,	Very rarely	80	Mostly
Basal/lateral	Alternans or lacunar syndrome	Possibly headache	–	10	30

TRAUMATIC LESIONS OF THE NERVOUS SYSTEM

Traumatic lesions of the nervous system
Craniocerebral trauma: clinical grading

	Mild (Concussion---Cerebral contusion------)	Moderate	Severe
Unconsciousness	Up to 15 min	Up to 1 h	>1 h
Disordered consciousness (amnesia)	Up to 1 h	Up to 24 h	>24 h
Neurological deficits	Rarely, always reversible	Rarely, often reversible	Frequent, often only partially reversible
Autonomic disorders	Rare	Frequent	Always
Brain oedema	–	Occasionally	Mostly
Subjective complaints	Regression within 3–4 days	Frequently regression. Lasting complaints may occur	Mostly persisting complaints

Indications for surgery after open and closed craniocerebral injury

Open craniocerebral trauma (breaching of CSF space)

Depressed fracture with dural tear: always operate

Anterior fossa fracture with CSF rhinorrhoea: always operate

Middle fossa (petrous) fracture with ear-drum damage and CSF otorrhoea: operate only if persistence > 1 week

Intracranial air in plain X-rays or CT: danger of ascending infection.

Closed craniocerebral trauma

Depressed fracture without dural tear or scalp laceration: operate only if depression as great as vault thickness, or greater

Skull-base fracture without breaching of CSF space, often with mono- or biorbital haematoma: no operation

Operation occasionally indicated for haematoma in middle ear, bleeding ear or nose

Traumatic intracranial bleeding

	Frequency in craniocerebral trauma (%)	Affected vessels(s)	Associated lesions	Operation	Mortality (%)
Acute subdural haematoma	10	Subdural veins	Always brain lesion	Trephining	60
Chronic subdural haematoma	10	Subdural veins	Head trauma, no associated lesion	Burr-holes, drainage	10
Extradural haematoma	1	Middle meningeal artery, venous sinus in posterior fossa	Temporal fracture	Trephining, ligation of artery	20
Intracerebral haematoma	25	Brain arteries	Invariably	Rarely, depending on location and size	50
Subarachnoid haemorrhage	10–20	Variable, an epiphenomenon	Always	None	Depends on other factors

Glasgow coma scale

(Reproduced after Teasdale, G. and Jennett, B. (1976) Assessment of coma and impaired consciousness. *Acta Neurochir (Wien)*, **34**, 45; *Lancet* (1974), **1**, 81–83.)

		Score
Eye opening	Spontaneously	4
	In response to speech	3
	In response to pain	2
	None	1
Verbal response	Orientated	5
	Confused	4
	Inappropriate, single words	3
	Incomprehensible sounds	2
	Absent	1
Motor responses	Obeys commands	6
	Localizing response to pain	5
	Flexor response to pain	4
	Atypical flexor response	3
	Extensor response	2
	Absent	1
Maximum score		15
Minimum score		3

Glasgow outcome scale

(Reproduced after Jennett, B. and Bond, M. (1975) Assessment of outcome after severe brain damage. *Lancet*, **1**, 480–484.)

1. Death without recovery of consciousness after brain trauma.
2. Persistent vegetative state: patient unresponsive, eyes open, vegetative functions intact.
3. Severe disability: patient conscious but disabled, requiring help because of physical and/or mental disability.
4. Moderate disability: patient manages daily activities (with aids), can use public transport and do sheltered work but has obvious disability.
5. Good recovery: resumption of normal life with slight neurological deficits.

Note:
- Record date of examination after date of trauma.
- Record details of physical and mental deficits.

The Glasgow outcome scale is also applicable for record of assessment after secondary brain damage (cardiac arrest, resuscitation), after encephalitis and strokes.

TRAUMATIC LESIONS OF THE NERVOUS SYSTEM

Clinical stages of craniocerebral trauma (a)

		Midbrain syndrome				Brain stem syndrome	
		I	II	III	IV	I	II
Consciousness		Drowsy	Coma	Coma	Coma	Coma	Coma
Response to	Noise	Adversion	Absent	Absent	Absent	Absent	Absent
	Pain	Localizing	Aimless	Flexion	Extension	Trace of extension	Absent
Ocular responses	Globes	Normal	Wobble	Diverge	Diverge	Fixed divergence	Fixed divergence
	Pupils	Medium	Medium	Constricted	Slightly constricted ↓↓	Dilated	Dilated, irregular
	Light reaction	Brisk	↓	↓	Absent	Absent	Absent
Brain stem reflexes	Oculocephalic*	Limited	Doll's eye +	Doll's eye +	Limited (+)	Absent	Absent
	Cilospinal	+	+	Cold stimulus: ipsilateral tonic response	Only ipsilateral	Absent	Absent
	Vestibulo-ocular (caloric)**	+	+			Absent	Absent
Somatic motor activity	Posture	Normal	Legs extended	Upper limbs flexed, lower limbs extended	Extension	Extension	Flaccidity
	Tone	Normal	Lower limbs increased		Extensor spasms	↑	Flaccid
	Spontaneous mobility	Mass movements	Mass movements of upper limbs	Flexor and extensor spasms	Extensor spasms	(extensor spasms)	–
	Babinski	–	(+)	+	+	(+)	–
Respiration and autonomic state	Breathing	Irregular	Possibly Cheyne-Stokes periodicity	↑	Hyperactive panting	↓	Absent
	Pulse rate	(↑)	(↑)	↑	↑↑	(↑)	↑
	Blood pressure	Normal	(↑)	↑	↑↑	(↑)	↑
	Temperature	Normal		↑	↑↑	(↑)	Normal ↓

*Test only when cervical spine injury has been excluded
**Test only when ear drums are intact

Clinical stages of craniocerebral trauma (b)

(Reproduced after Lücking, C.H. (1976) Klinische Stadien des Schädel-Hirn-Traumas, *Intensivbehandlung*, **1**, 26.)

Stages of brain disorder	Midbrain syndrome				Brainstem syndrome	
	1	2	3	4	1	2
Vigilance	Drowsy	Stupor	Coma	Coma	Coma	Coma
Response to sensory stimuli	Delayed	Reduced	Absent	Absent	Absent	Absent
Spontaneous motor activity						
Motor response to pain						
Muscle tone	Normal	Increased in lower limbs	Increased	Greatly increased	Normal – flaccid	Flaccid
Pupil size						
Pupil light reaction						
Eye movements	Pendular	Dysconjugate	Absent	Absent	Absent	Absent
Oculocephalic reflex		+	++	+Ø	Ø	Ø
Caloric vestibulo-ocular response	Normal ++		Tonic	Dissociated		
Respiration						
Temperature	Normal	Normal	Slightly raised	Greatly raised	Reduced	Greatly reduced
Pulse rate						
Blood pressure						

TRAUMATIC LESIONS OF THE NERVOUS SYSTEM

Cranial nerve damage from trauma

Nerve(s)	Consequence	Mechanism	Treatment	Prognosis
Olfactory (filaments)	Anterior fossa fracture, blunt head trauma, contusions	Stretch/rupture of filaments (neuronal), cerebral contusion (central)	None	Spontaneous recovery up to 1 year, then poor
Optic	Fracture of orbit, optic canal, middle fossa	Contusion, haematoma	Operative decompression	Dependent on surgery, variable
Oculomotor	Orbital, craniofacial fracture, severe craniocerebral trauma	Direct or indirect pressure damage	Corticosteroids	Variable
Trochlear	Orbital fracture	Direct or indirect pressure damage	Corticosteroids	Variable
Trigeminal	Craniofacial, orbital and petrous fractures	Direct pressure damage	Surgery for mandibular lesion, otherwise corticosteroids	Variable
Abducens	Orbital fracture, severe craniocerebral trauma	Direct or indirect pressure damage	Corticosteroids	Variable
Facial	Laterobasal fractures	Immediate stretching, late compression by oedema, haemorrhage	Surgery for immediate palsy, if delayed corticosteroids, expectant	Dependent on surgery, variable
Vestibulocochlear	Laterobasal fractures, cerebral contusion	Petrous fracture site may produce middle or inner ear deafness, direct VIII nerve lesion	Surgery for middle ear deafness not for inner ear	Favourable, irreversible
Glossopharyngeal and vagus	Posterior fossa fractures	Pressure lesions	None	Variable
Spinal-accessory	Neck lesions	Direct lesion	Possibly graft operation	Irreversible
Hypoglossal	Hypoglossal foramen fracture	Compression in canal	Surgical decompression	Unfavourable

199

The risk of epilepsy after head injuries

(Reproduced after Glötzner, S. (1976) Post-traumatische Epilepsie. *Fortschr Med*, **94**, 1027–1031. Also Jennett, B. *Epilepsy After Non-Missile Head Injuries*, published by Heinemann, London, 1975.)

Type of injury	Epilepsy risk (%)
Closed injury (dura intact)	
Moderate craniocerebral trauma (disordered consciousness up to 24 h)	5
Severe craniocerebral trauma (disordered consciousness >24 h)	≤10
Uncomplicated linear or depressed skull fracture	≤10
After early post-traumatic epilepsy (in first week)	30
Depressed fracture with disordered consciousness >24 h or early epilepsy	50
Open trauma (dural tear)	
Penetrating brain injury (stab, bullet) without disorder of consciousness or early epilepsy	20
Open depressed or linear fracture	30
Dural tear with neurological deficit	50
Combined dural-brain lesion with complication (bleed, infection)	60

Indications for anticonvulsant prophylaxis after craniocerebral trauma

(treatment for 2 years)
1. Early epilepsy (20% frequency after severe craniocerebral trauma).
2. Depressed fracture with amnesia >24 h or EEG focus.
3. Acute subdural or extradural haematoma.
4. Open craniocerebral injuries.

Frequency of late (>3 months) post-traumatic epilepsy

Altogether up to 10% of medium and severe craniocerebral injuries.

Manifestation: up to end of first year after trauma in 50%
up to end of second year after trauma in 94%
up to end of tenth year after trauma: annual risk about 1%, thereafter annual risk <0.3%

TRAUMATIC LESIONS OF THE NERVOUS SYSTEM

Differential diagnosis of inability to establish contact with a 'wakeful' patient

Persistent vegetative state	Locked-in syndrome	Akinetic mutism
Cerebral hemispheres affected	Brain stem affected	Subfrontal brain damage, hemispheres intact elsewhere
Midbrain and brain stem intact	Cerebral hemispheres intact	Brain stem intact
Fixed body posture and motor automatism	Loss of all voluntary mobility except vertical eye movements	Marked lack of 'drive', with lack of all reactivity and responsiveness
Eyes open, do not fix, primitive reflexes elicitable, no reaction to environment	Sensory and special sensory pathways intact	Only discrete responses to painful stimuli. Patient capable of spontaneous speech and movement
Preserved sleep–wake rhythm with increased sympathetic tone	EEG intact	Incontinence, primitive reflexes may be elicited
Diffuse bilateral cerebral hemisphere damage	Bilateral pontine lesion	Bilateral subfrontal brain damage

Criteria of brain death

(Reproduced after Bundesaerztekammer *Dtsch Aerztebl*, **83**, 2940–2946 (1986); *Dtsch Aerztebl*, 2855–2860 (1991).)

Mandatory exclusions

- Intoxications
- Use of relaxant and sedative drugs
- Primary hypothermia
- Hypovolaemic shock
- Metabolic coma
- Endocrine coma
- Brain stem encephalitis
- Neuromuscular blockade.

Clinical neurological examination by two independent observers

Coma

No spontaneous respiration (apnoea test at arterial $pCO_2 > 50\,mmHg$)

Pupils medium or fully dilated and unreactive to light

Oculocephalic reflex absent (doll's eye phenomenon)

Absent corneal reflex in both eyes

No reaction to trigeminal pain (pricking nasal septum).

Period of observation

In adults: 12 h after primary brain damage

In children: 72 h after secondary brain damage; always at least 24 h

In premature infants and neonates (up to 4th week): always 72 h, plus obligatory EEG.

Note: multimodal evoked potentials (EP) not applicable in children.

Criteria of brain death in different countries

(Reproduced after Frowein, R.A. *et al.* (1985) Probleme des Hirntodes. *Verh Dtsch Ges Neurol*, **3**, 543–553.)

	Germany 1991	USA 1981	UK 1976	Switzerland 1983
Preconditions				
Diagnosis	+	+	+	+
No intoxication	+	+	+	+
normothermia	+	+	+	+
normovolemia	+	+	+	+
Clinical findings				
Coma	+	+	+	+
Apnoea test	+	+	+	+
(pCO$_2$ mmHg)	>60	>60	>50	>50
Fixed dilated pupils	+	+	+	+
Absent brain stem reflexes	+	+	+	+
Number of examiners	2	1	2	1
Duration of observations (h)				
In primary brain damage	12	12	6	6
In secondary brain damage	72	24	12	48
Additional investigations				
EEG flat	30 min	6 h/30 min	–	×2 in 24 h
Auditory evoked potentials absent	+	–	–	–
Circulatory arrest	Angiography	Scintigraphy	–	Angiography
ICP over systolic BP	–	–	–	+

Additional investigations

1. **EEG**
   Isoelectric for 30 min at double amplification, time constant 1.5. Obligatory in primary infratentorial brain damage.
2. **Auditory evoked potentials**
   Absence of potentials III–V (I preserved bilaterally, or serial tests).
3. **Median nerve SSEP**
   Absence of response above cervical cord level (if cord or peripheral nerve damage have been excluded; serial testing).
4. **Transcranial Doppler sonography**
   Biphasic flow or early systolic low peaks <50 cm/s in middle cerebral arteries, internal carotids, basilar; serial testing: intervals ≥30 min.
5. **Radioperfusion scintigraphy**
   Absence of intracranial filling with normality elsewhere.
6. **Arterial digital subtraction angiography (DSA)**
   Visualization of carotid arch and both carotids.

MEMORIX NEUROLOGY

Disorders of the spinal cord
Cord transection at different levels: clinical features and orthotic measures

Level of lesion	Functional abilities	Provision of aids
(Innervation of marker muscle)	(a) Bodily care (b) Hand functions (c) Wheel-chair dependency, possibilities of locomotion (d) Training to stand or walk	
C3/4 (diaphragm)	(a) Totally care dependent (c) Mobile in electric wheel-chair (d) Standing with electrodynamic appliance	Electric wheel-chair with special (e.g. chin) controls, mechanical wheel-chair, hoist
C4/5 (biceps)	(a) Mainly care dependent (b) Eating and writing with appliances (c) Limited and level locomotion by mechical/electric wheel-chair (d) Standing with electrohydraulic aid	Electric/mechanical wheel-chair Writing aids for electric typewriter Electrohydraulic standing aid
C5/6 (extensor carpi radialis)	(a) Upper limbs limited independence (b) Eating and writing feasible (c) Uneven ground wheel-chair use, adapted motor vehicle (d) Standing with electrohydraulic aid	Electric/mechanical wheel-chair Writing aids for electric typewriter Electrohydraulic standing aid special upper limb controlled motor vehicle
C6/7 (triceps muscle)	(a) Mainly independent (b) Hand function (c) Lomotion possibilities, v.s. (C5/6) (d) Standing with appliance	Mechanical wheel-chair for aids, v.s. (C5/6) Electrohydraulic or mechanical standing appliance Special upper limb controlled motor vehicle
C7/8 (finger flexors and extensors, latissimus dorsi muscles)	(a) Independent of nursing care (c) Wheel-chair at large, adapted motor vehicle (d) Standing with appliance and upper limb props	Mechanical wheel-chair Electric typewriter, orthotic bars, props* Standing appliance, hand controlled motor vehicle
T1–9 (intercostals)	(c) Wheel-chair dependent (d) Training with props (parallel bars)	Mechanical wheel-chair, props*, standing and walking frame Hand controlled motor vehicle
T11/L2 (trunk muscles)	(c) Wheel-chair dependent (d) Walking with props (forearm supports), stairs feasible	Mechanical wheel-chair, props*, forearm crutches, hand controlled motor vehicle
L3/4 (quadriceps and tibialis anterior)	(c) Partly independent of wheel-chair (d) Walking with props (forearm supports), stairs feasible	Mechanical wheel-chair Props* without knee-locking, ankle calliper, forearm support, hand controlled motor vehicle
L5/S1 (hamstrings and peronei)	(c) Independent of wheelchair, walking with ankle splinting, mostly without upper limb props	Optional wheel-chair, ankle splints, orthopaedic shoes
S2/3	(c) Good mobility	

* Props: plastic splints, metal calipers (some with springs, knee-locking, etc.)
Note: cord transection invariably means bowel and bladder paralysis; at higher levels, in addition respiratory impairment.

DISORDERS OF THE SPINAL CORD

Spinal cord syndromes: anatomical patterns

Anterior spinal artery syndrome
Spinal cord infarction from occlusion of anterior spinal artery
Transverse cord lesion with posterior column sparing, causing dissociated sensory loss (deep sensations spared) and spastic paralysis below level of lesion, flaccid paralysis at lesion level, plus bowel and bladder paralysis.

Posterior spinal cord circulation syndrome (radicular arteries)
Posterior column ischaemia
Incomplete transection motor and sensory syndrome, with emphasis on deficit of deep sensations.

Extramedullary space occupying lesions
Ascending ipsilateral disorder of all sensory modalities with paraesthesiae, contralateral dissociated sensory disturbance, ipsilateral lower limb spastic palsy; later sensori-motor spastic paraplegia with sphincter involvement. Hyperpathia and pain at level of lesion, also flaccid paralysis if situated in front of cord.

Intramedullary space occupying lesion
Variable bilateral dissociated sensory disturbances, flaccid paresis at level of lesion, sphincter disturbances and spastic paraparesis below level of lesion.

Brown–Séquard syndrome
Hemicord lesion: ipsilateral spastic paresis and loss of deep sensations below lesion level with contralateral superficial sensory loss (dissociated); possibly radicular pain and flaccid paresis ipsilaterally at level of lesion.

Anterior spinal artery perforating branch lesion
Brown–Séquard syndrome of vascular origin.

Spinal cord transection syndrome
Flaccid paraplegia at onset, then spastic. Sensory loss of all modalities below lesion level, sphincter paralysis, flaccid paresis and hyperpathia at lesion level.

Conus medullaris, epiconus and cauda equina syndromes

1. **Conus medullaris syndrome (in cord from S3 down)**
   (a) Lesion at level of first lumbar vertebra
   (b) Saddle anaesthesia
   (c) Bladder and rectum paralysis (bladder overflow-incontinence, faecal incontinence)
   (d) Anal and bulbocavernosus reflexes absent (often concurrent radicular defects from lesions of adjacent cauda equina roots L3–S1).
2. **Epiconus syndrome (in cord from L4 to S2)**
   (a) Spinal cord transection at spinal level of thoracolumbar junction
   (b) Paresis or paralysis of hip extension and external rotation, of knee flexion and of feet and toes
   (c) Absence of ankle jerks
   (d) Disorder of sensation from L4 down
   (e) Paralysis of sphincters.
3. **Cauda equina syndrome**
   (a) Multiple root lesions below level of body of second lumbar vertebra
   (b) Saddle anaesthesia
   (c) Bladder and bowel paralysis (in complete cauda equina syndrome)
   (d) Segmental pareses below knees, possibly also knee flexors and buttock muscles
   (e) Segmental sensory disturbance in legs below knees and in feet
   (f) Absence of ankle jerks.

MEMORIX NEUROLOGY

Non-traumatic acute transverse cord lesions: differential diagnosis

	Extramedullary	Intramedullary
Tumour		
Malignant	Metastases	Glioma
Benign	Chordoma	Ependymoma
Degenerative	Disc prolapse Unstable odontoid	
Inflammatory	Epidural abscess	Multiple sclerosis, herpes viruses, HIV, HTLV 1, enteroviruses, syphilis, vasculitides, parainfectious, inoculation reaction
Vascular	Haematoma	Ischaemia, haemorrhage, AV fistulae
Toxic		Drug abuse, radiation myelopathy

DISORDERS OF THE SPINAL CORD

Spinal dysrhaphism

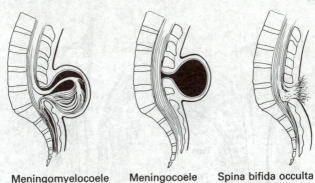

Meningomyelocoele   Meningocoele   Spina bifida occulta

Blood supply of spinal cord

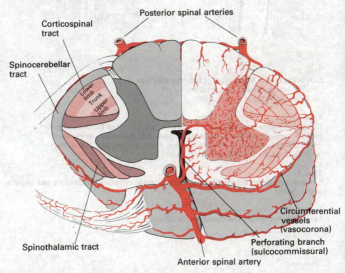

Types of Arnold – Chiari malformations

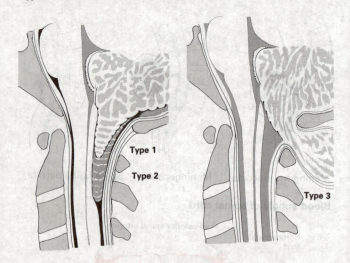

Type 1
Cerebellar tonsils below level of foramen magnum
(in 50% syringomyelia, hydromyelia;
in 10% associated hydrocephalus).

Type 2
Cerebellar vermis, medulla and IV ventricle below level of foramen magnum
(in 90% syringomyelia, hydromyelia, Klippel–Feil syndrome, dysraphism;
in 80% hydrocephalus, aqueduct stenosis, other cerebral malformations;
in 10% associated malformations of viscera.)

Type 3
Cervico-occipital meningomyelocoele with inclusion of parts of cerebellum and medulla in the cavity.

Type 4
Cerebellar hypoplasia associated with malformation type 1, 2 and 3.

DISORDERS OF THE SPINAL CORD

Synopsis of diseases of the spinal cord

Clinical features	Upper motor neuron: cortico-spinal tracts	Lower motor neuron: anterior horn cells, bulbar nuclei	Posterior columns	Spinothalamic tracts	Spinocerebellar tracts
	Spastic paresis, pyramidal tract signs	Flaccid palsy with wasting, fasciculation	Lost deep sensations, sensory ataxia, dysaesthesiae	Contralateral pain and temperature loss	Hypotonia ataxia
Diseases					
Motor neuron disease	+	+	0	0	0
Hereditary spastic paraplegia	+	0	0	0	0
Spinal muscular atrophies	0	+	0	0	0
Subacute combined degeneration (B₁₂ deficiency)	(+)	0	+	0	0
Syringomyelia (s.-bulbia)	+	(+)	0	+	0
Friedreich's ataxia	(+)		+	0	+
Tabes dorsalis	(+)	(+)	+	0	0

Spinal muscular atrophies

Type	Eponym	Affected parts	Age of onset (years)	Heredity
Infantile proximal	Werdnig–Hoffmann	Generalized pseudohypertrophy and weakness, early respiratory involvement	0–2	Autosomal recessive
Chronic proximal form (pseudomyopathic)	Kugelberg–Welander	Pelvic girdle, shoulder girdle	3–18 (juvenile) 18–60 (adult)	Dominant or recessive (if recessive better prognosis)
Distal adult form	Aran–Duchenne	Fingers, arms, shoulders	30–50	Sporadic
Proximal adult form (scapulohumeral form)	Vulpian–Bernhardt	Shoulders, arms, hands	40–50	Sporadic
Scapuloperoneal form	–	Peronei, shoulders	30–40	Irregular
Progressive bulbar palsy	Fazio–Londe	Cranial nerves (VII, IX, X, XI, XII)	2–12	Sporadic
Peroneal form	–	Legs (below knees)	5–15	Irregular
Segmental forearm form	–	Unilateral: forearm and hand	20–25	Sporadic

Polyneuropathies
Causes of polyneuropathy in neurological practice

Alcohol	20–40%
Diabetes mellitus	15–30%
Guillain–Barré syndrome	6–13%
Tick-borne radiculopathy	up to 10%
Hereditary neuropathies	up to 5%
Paraneoplastic	up to 4%
Parainfectious	up to 3%
Malabsorption	up to 3%
Toxic substances	up to 3%
Vasculitis	up to 2%
Renal failure related	up to 2%
Multifactorial or unclassifiable	10–30%

Diagnostic strategies in polyneuropathy
(Reproduced after Berlit, P. *Klinische Neurologie*, published by VCH, Weinheim, 1992.)

Blood tests
ESR → vasculitis, tumour, para-/dysproteinaemias, rheumatoid disease
Transaminases → alcohol, toxic causes
Glucose (tolerance test), HbA1 → diabetes mellitus
Renal function tests → renal failure
T3, T4, TSH → thyroid diseases
Borrelia antibodies → borrelioses
Protein and immunoelectrophoresis → para-/dysproteinaemia, immunovasculitis
Antinuclear factors, serological tests for rheumatoid diseases → SLE, rheumatoid arthritis
Hepatitis serology → hepatitis, polyarteritis nodosa
Vitamin B12, folate → subacute combined degeneration of cord
Virology (herpes, enteroviruses, CMV, polio, mycoplasma) → viral/parainfectious polyneuritis
Angiotensin converting enzyme, lysozyme → sarcoidosis
Phytanic acid → Refsum's disease
Trihexosyl ceramidase → Fabry's disease (angiokeratoma corporis diffusum)
Toxins → tetanus, botulism, diphtheria
G_{M1} antibody → motor neuropathy with proximal conduction block.

Other investigations
Neurophysiology (neurography, EMG, SSEP, magnetic stimulation), autonomic function tests
CSF (Guillain–Barré syndrome, borrelioses)
Schilling test (subacute combined degeneration of cord)
Tuberculin test, gallium scintigram (sarcoidosis)
X-rays of chest and spine (sarcoidosis, myelomatosis)
Peripheral nerve biopsy (hereditary and toxic neuropathies, vasculitis, amyloidosis, etc.)
Rectal biopsy (amyloidosis).
Urinary porphobilinogen, δ-amino-laevulinic acid → porphyria

POLYNEUROPATHIES

Aetiology of polyneuritis and polyneuropathy

Polyneuritis caused by pathogenic agents
- Varicella – zoster virus
- AIDS
- Herpes simplex virus
- Leprosy
- Borrelia burgdorferi (Lyme disease)
- Trypanosomiasis

Immunologically mediated polyneuritis
1. Monoclonal gammopathies (primarily with plasmacytoma, Waldenström's macroglobulinaemia, cryoglobulinaemia; secondarily with lymphomas, amyloidosis, chronic inflammation, benign form).
2. Idiopathic (Guillain–Barré syndrome).
3. Miller–Fisher syndrome (ophthalmoplegia, ataxia, areflexia).
4. Para- and postinfectious in viral illnesses (CMV, Epstein–Barr, Varicella-zoster, mycoplasma pneumoniae, ECHO viruses, Coxsackie, enteroviruses, influenza, measles, rubella, mumps, hepatitis, dengue fever).
5. Postvaccinial (localized by injection site).
6. Serological (localized by injection site).
7. Pan-dysautonomia: motor polyneuritis with multifocal proximal conduction block (ganglioside antibody).
8. Paraneoplastic (carcinoma of bronchus, breast, gastrointestinal tract).
9. Neuralgic amyotrophy (syndrome of Parsonage and Aldren Turner).
10. Polyradiculitis of cauda equina (Elsberg syndrome).
11. Idiopathic neuritis of lumbosacral plexus.
12. Para- and postinfectious in bacterial illnesses (typhoid, paratyphoid, dysentery, scarlet fever, leptospirosis, brucellosis, rickettsial diseases).

Granulomatous-inflammatory neuropathy
- Melkersson–Rosenthal's syndrome (facial nerve)
- Sarcoidosis (cranial nerves).

Bacterial toxins as cause of neuropathy
- Diphtheria
- Botulism.

Metabolic polyneuropathy
- Uraemic
- Hepatic failure
- Primary biliary cirrhosis
- Malabsorption
- Wilson's disease
- Malnutrition
- Vitamin deficiencies
- Beri-beri
- Pellagra
- Hyperlipidaemia
- Oxalosis
- Haemochromatosis
- Porphyria
- Alcohol abuse.

Endocrine neuropathies
- Acromegaly
- Hypothyroidism (VIII nerve)
- Hyperthyroidism
- Multiple endocrine neoplasia
- Diabetes mellitus
- Hyperparathyroidism.

Vascular polyneuropathy
- Microangiopathy (diabetic)
- Hypersensitivity angiitis (amphetamine, penicillin, heroin)
- Ischaemic (arteriosclerosis, thromboangiitis obliterans)
- Polyarteritis nodosa
- Churg – Strauss syndrome (allergic granulomatosis)
- Systemic lupus erythematosus
- Rheumatoid arthritis
- Sjögren's disease
- Giant cell arteritis
- Scleroderma
- Syphilis.

Mechanically determined (pressure) neuropathies
- Arthropathies (including gout)
- Pregnancy
- Anticoagulation
- Tumours
- Coma (including general anaesthesia).

Toxic polyneuropathies

(Seaton, A. (1992) Organic solvents and the nervous system. *Quarterly Journal of Medicine*, **84**, 637–639.)

Organic solvents
Carbon disulphide, benzene, methyl alcohol (optic neuropathy), hexacarbons (phenol, white spirit, toluene, xylol: autonomic dysfuntion), carbon tetrachloride (incling optic nerve), tetrachloro-ethane (dysgeusia, small hand and foot muscles), trichloro-ethylene (trigeminal anaesthesia and dysaesthesiae), tetra-chloro-ethylene, chloro-bi-phenyl, mono-chloro-methane (visual disorder and ptosis), hydrazine, tri-ortho-cresyl-phosphate (mainly motor and autonomic, later also myelopathy), di-chloro-benzol (dysaesthesiae, optic nerve), acrylamide (mainly upper limbs, with rashes), ethylene oxide (peroneal palsy), dimethyl-amino-proprio-nitrile (early bladder and potency disorders, perianal sensory loss), phenol (median).

Pesticides, heavy metals, disinfectants
Arsenic (alopecia, pigmentation, hyperkeratosis, pains), barium polysulphide (purely motor), DDT (optic and acoustic nerve damage), di-nitro-phenol, mono-bromo-methane, phosphoric acid ester (long latency, myelopathy), penta-chloro-phenol (dysaesthesiae, possibly optic nerve), dichloro-phenoxy-acetic acid, thallium (hyperpathia, pelvic girdle, autonomic symptoms), di-chloro-benzene, lead (wrist drop), gold, mercury (mainly sensory), hexa-chlorophen, alkyl-phosphate (E600 and E605: motor, autonomic, myelopathy).

Polyneuropathies from drugs and medications

Chemotherapeutic agents, antibiotics, fungicides
Sulphonamides, dapsone (motor), nitrofurantoin (vitamin B_1 and B_6 deficiency), nitrofurazone (pain), furaltadone (cranial nerve involvement), hydroxyquinoline (optic nerve involvement, myelopathy), chloroquine (myopathy), diamines (trigeminal involvement), vidarabin (burning feet), metronidazole (sensory), ethambutol (optic nerve), ethionamide (sensory, reversible), isoniazid (vitamin B_6 deficiency, autonomic involvement), amphotericin B (motor), chloramphenicol (sensory, reversible, vitamin B_1 deficiency), gentamycin (VIII nerve damage), streptomycin (VIII nerve damage), polymyxin.

Cardiovascular drugs, anticoagulants
Amiodarone (reversible, paraesthesiae), hydralazine (vitamin B_6 deficiency), ergotamine derivatives (reversible), methysergide, disopyramide, sodium cyanate, phenytoin, clofibrate.

Psychotropic agents, sedatives, hypnotics
Amitriptyline (peroneal palsy), imipramine, phenelzine, lithium, thalidomide (dysaesthesiae), glutethimide, nitrous oxide (paraesthesiae, myelopathy).

Various drugs
Indomethacin, gold (pain), colchicine, phenytoin, disulfiram (dysaesthesiae, optic nerve involvement), cimetidine (reversible), carbamazepine, thiouracil derivatives (smell and taste disorders), carbimazole (smell and taste disorders), sulphonyl ureas: chlorpropamide, tolbutamide.

Cytostatic agents
Chlorambucil, nitrofurazone, vincristine (intestinal symptoms, cranial nerve involvement), vinblastin (reversible), cytarabine (sensory, reversible), procarbazine (sensory, reversible), cis-platinum (ototoxicity, optic nerve damage).
Local infusion nerve damage: mustine, melphalan, dactinomycin (actinomycin D).

POLYNEUROPATHIES

Hereditary polyneuropathies

(Reproduced after Harding, A. and Thomas, P.K. (1984) in *Peripheral Nerve Disorders*, (eds Asbury, A. and Gilliat, R.), Butterworth, London.)

	Mode of inheritance / Age of onset	Characteristics
Hereditary motor and sensory neuropathies (HMSN) Neural muscular atrophies		
Neurogenic muscular atrophy of Charcot, Marie, Tooth demyelinating hypertrophic form (HMSN type I)	Autosomal dominant or X-linked chromosome, age 10–30 years	Thickened nerves, areflexia Polyneuropathic syndrome
Axonal, neuronal form (HMSN type II)	Autosomal dominant or recessive, age 25–40 years	Distal polyneuropathic syndrome
Hypertrophic neuropathy of Dejerine–Sottas (HMSN type III)	Autosomal recessive, up to 10th year, M:F = 2:1	Thickened nerves, polyneuropathic syndrome, cranial nerves involved, rapid progression
Hereditary sensory neuropathies (HSN)		
Mutilating neuropathies (HSN type I)	Autosomal dominant, youth	Pain, ulceration, analgesia
Infantile sensory neuropathy (HSN type II)	Autosomal recessive, infants	Mainly upper limbs, areflexia, ulceration
Familial dysautonomia Riley–Day (HSN type III)	Autosomal recessive, congenital	Dysphagia, vomiting, corneal ulcers
Swanson syndrome (HSN type IV)	Autosomal recessive, congenital	Analgesia, anhidrosis
Other hereditary polyneuropathies		
Congenital general imperception of pain	Autosomal recessive, sporadic, infantile	Anhidrosis
Hereditary neuropathy with liability to pressure palsies	Autosomal dominant, all ages	Recurrent pressure palsies
Giant axonal neuropathy	Autosomal recessive, infantile	Polyneuropathic syndrome, gait disorder, areflexia, cranial nerve symptoms
Cerebellar ataxia with spinal muscular atrophy	Autosomal dominant, infantile	Cerebellar signs, muscular atrophy, lower cranial nerves
Cerebellar ataxia with neurogenic muscular atrophy	Autosomal recessive, infantile	Cerebellar signs, skeletal deformities
Hereditary synkinesia (mirror movements)	Irregular dominant, congenital M:F = 2:1	Bilateral syndrome, voluntary movements
Neurogenic muscular atrophy + essential tremor (Roussy–Levy syndrome)	Autosomal dominant, infantile	Slow progression, motor, gait ataxia, areflexia

Hereditary polyneuropathies with metabolic and other defects

	Mode of inheritance, age of onset	Clinical features
Hereditary amyloid neuropathies		
Portuguese type	Autosomal dominant 20th–40th year	Rapid progression to death
Indiana type		Worse lower limbs, viscera affected
Iowa (van Allen) type		Worse upper limbs, eyes involved
Finnish type		Diffuse, kidneys involved
		Cranial polyneuropathy
Neuropathies with disorders of lipid metabolism		
Hereditary high density lipoprotein deficiency (Tanger disease)	Autosomal recessive, any age	Various types of manifestation
Abeta-lipoproteinaemia (Bassen–Kornzweig disease)	Autosomal dominant, or infantile recessive	Acanthocytosis, areflexia, pyramidal tract signs
Phytanic acid storage disease (Refsum's disease)	Autosomal recessive, up to age 30 years	Retinitis pigmentosa, deafness, cerebellar signs, cardiomyopathy
Angiokeratoma corporis diffusum (Fabry's disease) (alpha-galactosidase A deficiency)	X chromosome, recessive	Pain, dysaesthesiae, analgesia
Metachromatic leucodystrophy (sulphatide lipidosis) (aryl-sulphatase A deficiency)	Autosomal recessive, any age	Dementia, cerebellar signs, spasticity
Adrenomyeloneuropathy and leucodystrophy	Autosomal recessive, infantile	Spasticity, bladder disorders, Addison's disease
Globoid cell leucodystrophy (Krabbe's disease) (galactosyl-ceramide lipidosis)	Autosomal recessive, infantile	Epilepsy, blindness
Cockayne syndrome	Autosomal recessive, infantile	Dwarfism, areflexia, dementia, cerebellar signs, eyes and ears involved
Cerebrotendinous xanthomatosis	Autosomal recessive, infantile	Dementia, spasticity, cerebellar, sensory, cataracts
Hereditary porphyrias		
Acute intermittent porphyria	Autosomal dominant, 20–40 years	Colicky abdominal pains
Variegate porphyria		Photosensitivity of skin
Hereditary coproporphyria		Colicky abdominal pains, cranial nerve deficits

POLYNEUROPATHIES

Guillain–Barré syndrome: definition

(Reproduced after Asbury, A.K. *et al.* (1978) Criteria for diagnosis of Guillain–Barré syndrome. *Annals of Neurology*, **3**, 565.)

> Progressive motor and mainly symmetrical peripheral nervous system disorder, usually maximal within 4 weeks from onset
>
> +
>
> Areflexia
>
> +
>
> Slowed nerve conduction velocities (<70%) on neurophysiological testing (often patchy or proximal conduction block)
>
> and / or
>
> Reduction of amplitudes (<80%)
>
> +
>
> CSF protein increase + normal cells after first week
>
> Improvement starts 2–4 weeks after symptomatic peale
>
> **Optional features**
>
> Cranial nerve involvment (facial nerve in 50%)
>
> Sensory symptoms/signs
>
> Disorders of autonomic functions
>
> CSF pleocytosis
>
> Absence of CSF protein rise
>
> Normal neurophysiology initially (in up to 15%)

Chronic inflammatory demyelinating polyneuritis (CIDP): definition

(Reproduced after American Academy of Neurology (1991) Criteria of CIDP. *Neurology*, **41**, 617.)

Progressive or relapsing motor and sensory dysfunction of more than one limb of a peripheral nerve nature over at least 2 months, plus hypo- or areflexia, reduction in conduction velocities <70%, and/or amplitude reduction <80%.

CSF protein raised, with cell count <10/mm^3 if HIV negative, or <50 if HIV positive.

Diet in phytanic acid storage (Refsum's) disease

(Reproduced from Neundörfer, B. *Polyneuritiden and Polyneuropathien*, published by VCH, Weinheim, 1987.)

	Allowed	Prohibited
Fats	Vegetable fats	Butter, lard, bacon
Milk products	Skim milk, low fat cheese, yoghurt	Ice cream, cream, unskimmed milk, high and medium fat cheese
Meat and fish	Lean veal and beef, venison, lean fish, lean ham, non-fatty soup, lean poultry	Fatty meat and fish, goose, duck, sardines, sausages
Eggs		All foods containing egg yolks, mayonnaise
Fruit	Peeled apple and pears, oranges, tangerines, grapefruit, banana, peach, apricot, pineapple	Grapes, unpeeled apple and pear
Vegetables	Carrots, cauliflower, celery, asparagus, beetroot, turnip, kohlrabi, fennel, radishes	Green beans, peas, broccoli, cabbages, sprouts, lettuce, endives, cucumber, parsley, leeks, green pepper, spinach
Desserts and sweets	Cakes and pastries prepared with vegetable margarine and few eggs, jams, honey, sugar	Chocolate, cocoa, ovaltine
Nuts		All types of nuts
Bread	All types of bread	
Accompaniments	Rice, potato, pastry (low egg yolk)	

Varieties of immunoneuropathy

- Acute polyradiculopathy (Guillain–Barré syndrome)
- Polyradiculitis (chronic inflammatory demyelinating polyneuritis: CIDP)
- Neuropathy with gammopathies
  (a) With benign gammopathy
  (b) With myeloma
  (c) With macroglobulinaemia (Waldenström's syndrome)
  (b) With primary amyloidosis
- Motor neuron syndromes (motor neuron disease, G_{M1} neuropathy, post-poliomyelitis syndrome)
- Paraneoplastic neuropathies
- Pathogen-induced neuropathies (e.g. with HIV infection, borreliosis)
- Systemic and non-systemic vasculitides

POLYNEUROPATHIES

Features of autonomic involvment in polyneuropathy

(may occur in diabetes mellitus, Guillain–Barré syndrome, porphyria, amyloidosis, toxic neuropathies, e.g. alcohol, INH, lead, uraemia, hereditary neuropathies)

	Symptoms	Diagnostic tests
Cardiovascular	Tachycardia at rest Silent infarction	ECG: variability of rate on hyperventilation, Valsalva manoeuvre, drugs (atropine, beta-blockade)
	Orthostatic hypotension	BP responses on standing
Gastrointestinal	Nocturnal diarrhoea	Small bowel biopsy (to exclude coeliac disease, etc.)
	Distension, heartburn, dysphagia	Barium meal and follow-through, including timing of passage
	Undetected hypoglycaemia	Absence of insulin-induced tachycardia
	Pancreatic exocrine failure	Secretin-pancreozymin test
	Gallbladder distension and stones Salivary gland disease	Diagnostic ultrasound Palpation
Genitourinary	Impotence	Testicular compression painless
	Retrograde ejaculation Retention of urine (incomplete bladder emptying)	Urine microscopy Ultrasound, urodynamic tests
Trophic changes	Hypo-/anhidrosis of feet Vasomotor paralysis Trophic oedema, alopecia, painless ulceration, nail dystrophy	Sweat tests Histamine test (with noradrenaline) Galvanometric skin resistance tests (startle response) (EMG leads)
	Osteoarthropathy	Plain X-rays

There may be absence of obvious signs of polyneuropathy (reduced vibration sense, glove and stocking sensory impairment, loss of tendon jerks), i.e. a purely autonomic neuropathy

Primary screening tests are underlined
Reference: Bannister, R. (1988) *Autonomic Failure*, Oxford University Press, Oxford.

MEMORIX NEUROLOGY

Treatment possibilities of the causes of polyneuropathy

Alcoholic polyneuropathy (PNP)	Abstinence, vitamin B (thiamine)
Diabetic PNP	Good, but not extreme, diabetic control, Aldose reductase inhibitors
Guillain–Barré syndrome	Plasmapheresis 7S immunoglobulin (7S Ig)
CIDP (chronic inflammatory demyelinating PNP)	Corticosteroids, plasmapheresis, 7S Ig
Borreliosis (Lym disease)	Cephalosporins, tetracycline
Other polyneuritides	Specific (dapsone for leprosy, acyclovir for varicella-zoster virus, antitoxin for diphtheria)
Toxic PNP	Exclusion of toxic agents, possibly antidote
Paraproteinaemic PNP	Treatment of underlying disease (Waldenström's disease, myeloma), or plasmapheresis (for benign gammopathies)
PNP with Gm1 antibody	Cyclophosphamide
PNP with vasculitides, collagenoses	Corticosteroids, immunosuppressants (azathioprine, cyclophosphamide)
Uraemic PNP	Effective haemodialysis (duration rather than frequency of dialyses matters), renal transplant
Thyroid diseases	Correction of underlying disorder
Malabsorption, vitamin deficiencies	Correction of deficiencies
Refsum's disease	Low phytanic acid diet
Abeta-lipoproteinaemia	Low fat diet, vitamins A and E
Paraneoplastic polyneuropathy	Corticosteroids, immunosuppressants

PERIPHERAL NERVE LESIONS

Areas of referred pain (areas according to Henry Head)
(Reproduced after Hansen, K. and Schlack, H. *Segmental Innervation*, published by Thieme, Stuttgart, 1962.)

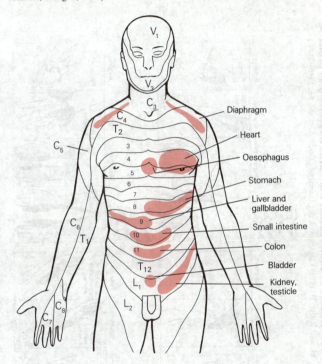

Syndromes of cervical spinal root compression from intervertebral disc prolapse

(Reproduced after Stöhr, M. and Riffel, B. (1989) Diagnostik der Ischialgie. *Dtsch Aerztebl*, 86, 1146–1149.)

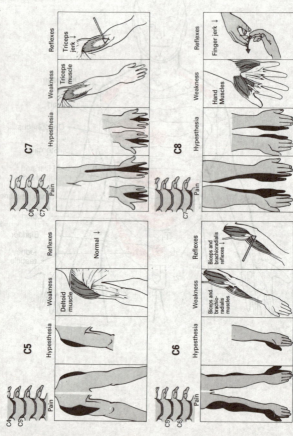

PERIPHERAL NERVE LESIONS

Syndromes of lumbosacral spinal root compression from intervertebral disc prolapse

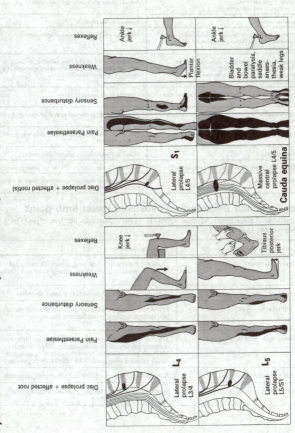

Causes of lumbosacral root disorders

(Reproduced after Stöhr, M. and Riffel, B. (1989) Diagnosis der Ischialgie. *Dtsch Aerztebl*, **86**, 1146–1149.)

Causes	Main localization and clinical features
Spinal degenerative changes (spondylosis and osteoarthritis)	Monoradicular syndromes, especially roots L4–S1
Lumbar stenosis	Neurogenic 'claudication'
Other spinal troubles (spondylolisthesis, ankylosing spondylitis, trauma, tumours, inflammations, osteoporosis with spontaneous fractures)	Unilateral and bilateral lesions of nerve roots
Tumours of nerve roots and adjacent structures (neurinoma, meningioma, sedondary carcinoma or sarcoma, plasmacytoma, lymphomas. Differential diagnosis: abscess, haematoma)	Initially unilateral painful root syndrome, spreading to polyradicular, bilateral or cauda equina syndrome (e.g. epidural tumour extension)
Localized lumbosacral tumourous malformation and ependymoma	Conus or cauda equina syndrome
Carcinomatous or sarcomatous meningitis and tumour metastases (medulloblastoma)	Polyradicular symptoms and signs (CSF cytology +)
Dysrhaphism and tethered cord syndrome	Conus-cauda equina syndromes, especially with growth spurts in children
Arachnoiditis	Mono- and polyradicular irritation and defects
Radiculitis (zoster, herpes simplex, Lym disease)	Appropriate skin rashes, CSF cells and protein raised
Metabolic radiculopathies	Chiefly in elderly diabetics: involvement single or multiple thoracic or lumbar roots

Non-radicular neurological causes of lower limb pains

(Reproduced after Stöhr, M. and Riffel, B. (1989) Diagnosis der Ischialgie. *Dtsch Aerztebl*, **86**, 1146–1149.)

Localization of disease process	Particular features
Central nervous system	Thalamic syndrome: intra- and extramedullary cord lesions (especially lumbosacral enlargement and conus medullaris)
Peripheral nervous system	Polyneuropathies and hereditary system disorders
Lumbosacral plexus	Pelvic and hip trauma, inflammations, tumour spread, late radiation effect, psoas haematoma or abscess, diabetes
Lower limb peripheral nerves	Trauma and surgical lesions, misdirected im injections; compression (meralgia paraesthetica, tarsal tunnel, Morton's metatarsalgia, saphenous nerve in adductor canal; external compression by bandaging or posture)
Compartment syndromes	Anterior and posterior tibial and other compartments
Autonomic nervous system	Sympathetic reflex dystrophy, tumour infiltration of lumbar sympathetic chain

PERIPHERAL NERVE LESIONS

Classification of peripheral nerve injuries
(Reproduced after Sutherland, S. (1952) A classification of nerve injuries producing loss of function. *Brain*, **75**, 19.)

Grade 1	Neurapraxia Conduction block from myelin sheath damage
Grade 2	Axonotmesis I Interruption of axon, distal Wallerian degeneration
Grade 3	Axonotmesis II Additional lesion of endoneurium
Grade 4	Axonotmesis III Additional lesion of perineurium
Grade 5	Neurontmesis Complete nerve transection including epineurium

Grades 4 and 5 constitute an absolute indication for surgical intervention

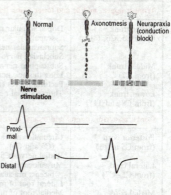

Differential diagnosis of brachial plexus from cervical root lesions

Brachial plexus	Cervical root
Histamine test negative (no flare) (intradermal injection 0.1 ml of 1/1000 solution of histamine)	Histamine test positive
Diminished sensory nerve action potential	Normal sensory nerve action potential
Hypo- or anhidrosis in area of reduced sensation	Increased or normal sweating in anaesthetic territory
EMG: normal in paravertebral muscles	EMG: paravertebral muscles show denervation (7–10 days)
Proximal neurography: infraganglionic type of defect (F-wave, SSEP)	Proximal neurography: supraganglionic type of defect
Myelography normal	Myelography may show empty or ruptured root pockets
CSF clear	CSF haemorrhagic
Invariably multiradicular	Monoradicular or multiradicular
No cervical pain syndrome	Cervical pain syndrome

MEMORIX NEUROLOGY

Brachial plexus lesions

Brachial plexus	Peripheral nerves
Trunks: upper, middle and lower trunk lesions	
Upper trunk (from C5, C6, C4)	Dorsal scapular nerve (to rhomboids and levator scapulae)
	Suprascapular nerve (to supra- and infraspinatus)
	Subclavian nerve (to subclavius)
Middle trunk (from C7)	Subscapular nerve (to subscapularis and teres major)
	Long thoracic nerve (to serratus anterior muscles)
	Pectoral nerves (to pectoralis major and minor muscles)
Lower trunk (from C8 and T1)	Thoracodorsal nerve (to latissimus dorsi)
Cords: posterior, lateral and medial cord lesions	
Posterior cord (from C5 to T1)	Circumflex nerve (to deltoid and teres minor muscles) (C5 and C6)
	Radial nerve (C5–T1)
Lateral cord (from C5–C7)	Musculocutaneous nerve (C5–C7) (to coracobrachialis, biceps, brachialis muscles)
	Lateral root of median nerve (C5–C7)*
Medial cord (from C8 and T1)	Medial root of median nerve (C8, T1)**
	Ulnar nerve (C8, T1)
	Medial cutaneous nerve of arm (C8, T1)
	Medial cutaneous nerve of forearm (C8, T1)

Upper plexus lesion (Erb – Duchenne)
Paresis of deltoid, supra- and infraspinatus, biceps, supinator and brachioradialis muscles
Sensory disturbance over deltoid and radial side of forearm (not invariably)
Biceps and brachioradialis (supinator) jerks absent

Middle plexus lesion (mostly in combination with upper plexus lesion)
Paresis of triceps, wrist and finger extensor, pronator teres muscles
Sensory disturbance radial side of hand and C7 dermatome
Loss of finger jerk

Lower plexus lesion (Dejerine – Klumpke)
Paresis of ulnar and median innervated small hand muscles (lumbricals, interossei, flexors)
Sensory disturbance ulnar border of forearm and hand
Loss of finger jerk
(Often associated homolateral Horner's syndrome from cervical sympathetic lesion)

* Pronator teres, flexor digitorum and pollicis longus muscles. Reduced sensation digits 1–3
** Thenar palsy without sensory loss

PERIPHERAL NERVE LESIONS

Brachial plexus: spinal root supply (C4–T1) and peripheral distribution
(Reproduced from Stöhr, M. and Riffel, B. *Nerven und Nervenwurzelläsionen*, published by VCH, Weinheim, 1988.) (illustration without nerves to shoulder muscles)

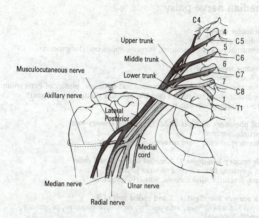

Main features of brachial plexus lesions

Upper plexus lesion (Erb – Duchenne); roots C5–C6
Paresis of shoulder abduction and external rotation and of elbow flexion. Biceps and superior jerks lost. Sensation lost from shoulder tip down to radial side of forearm.

Lower plexus lesion (Dejerine – Klumpke); roots C8–T1
Paresis of finger flexion and small hand muscles. Finger jerk absent
Sensory loss ulnar border of hand and forearm. Possible associated Horner's syndrome.

Middle plexus lesion; root C7 (uncommon, usually part of upper plexus lesion)
Paresis of arm, hand and finger extension. Triceps jerk absent
Sensory loss digits 2 and 3, extending strip up hand and forearm.

Main features of brachial plexus cord lesions
Posterior cord: axillary and radial nerves
Paresis of shoulder abduction, arm, hand and finger extension
Sensory disturbance lateral border of arm and forearm.

Lateral cord: musculocutaneous and lateral root of median nerve
Paresis of elbow flexion, pronation, wrist and finger flexion
Sensory disturbance digits 1 to 3, radial border of forearm.

Medial cord: ulnar and medial root of median nerve, medial cutaneous nerves of arm and forearm
Paresis of thenar muscles, finger adduction and abduction, ulnar flexion of wrist and fingers
Sensory disturbance in ulnar border of hand.

MEMORIX NEUROLOGY

Common causes of peripheral nerve lesions
(Expanded from Stöhr, M. and Riffel, B. *Nerven- und Nervenwurzelläsionen*, published by VCH, Weinheim, 1988.)

Causes of median nerve palsy

Palsy including pronator teres
Site of lesion: medial aspect of arm
'Lovers palsy' (nocturnal pressure), trauma, surgery, supracondylar process

Palsy without pronator teres involvement
Lesion at elbow (flexor aspect)
Instrumentation for angiography, etc., dislocations and fractures, plaster of Paris splint
Pronator teres syndrome, sublimis tunnel (tendon of flexor digitorum sublimis)
Bicipital aponeurosis (lacertus fibrosus)

Paresis of terminal phalanges of digits 1, 2, (3), without sensory loss
Site of lesion: proximal forearm
Anterior interosseous syndrome from compression by bands.

Thenar palsy with sensory loss digits 1, 2, radial half of 3 and palm
Lesion site: distal forearm, flexor aspect of wrist joint
Penetrating trauma, fractures, dislocations, surgery, injections.

Thenar palsy with sensory loss digits 1, 2 and radial half of 3
Site of lesion: carpal tunnel (fibrosis, arthropathy, repetitive pressure, pregnancy, acromegaly, hypothyroidism)
Sensory loss of whole, or halves, of digits 1–3
Site of lesion: palm
Penetrating injuries, plaster of Paris pressure.

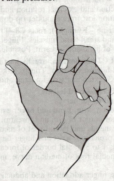

Posture making fist: thumb and index extended

PERIPHERAL NERVE LESIONS

Causes of ulnar nerve palsy

Palsy including flexion of terminal phalanx of digit 5 (medial half flexor digitorum profundus)
Lesion site: arm or elbow
Ulnar groove syndrome: late result of trauma, mobile and subluxating ulnar nerve, degenerative changes, pressure (e.g. plaster of Paris, crutches), tumours, surgery, trauma, cubital tunnel syndrome (aponeurosis distal to medial epicondyle).

Palsy with sensory loss ulnar border of hand on dorsal side (ramus dorsalis)
Lesion site: proximal forearm
Fractures, soft tissue injuries, A-V shunt operation (possibly dorsal ramus only).

Palsy of all ulnar supplied small hand muscles, sensory loss digits 5 and half of 4
Site of lesion: wrist joint
Penetrating injuries, tumours, narrowing of ulnar (or Guyon's) tunnel at wrist.

Isolated paralysis of interossei, lumbricals, adductor pollicis, flexor pollicis brevis (deep branch)
Site of lesion: palm
Cyclists palsy, ulnar (or Guyon's) tunnel, injuries to palm.

Isolated sensory loss in digits 5 and half of 4 (superficial branch)
Site of lesion: ulnar side of palm, ulnar (or Guyon's) tunnel.

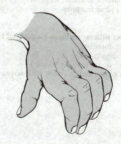

Claw hand

MEMORIX NEUROLOGY

Radial nerve lesions

Causes of radial nerve palsy

With paralysis of triceps muscle

Lesion site: in axilla
Crutch palsy, plaster of Paris cast.

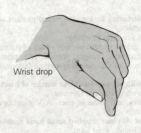
Wrist drop

With paralysis of brachioradialis muscle
Lesion site: arm above elbow
Fracture of shaft of humerus
'Saturday night' (park bench) palsy.

Wrist drop with sensory loss dorsum of hand (radial side)
Lesion site: elbow
Injuries, operations.

Paresis of finger extensors without sensory loss (deep branch)
Lesion site: proximal part of forearm
'Radial tunnel' syndrome, local lumps (ganglion, fibroma)
Displaced radius fractures.

Sensory loss without paralysis (superficial branch)
Lesion site: forearm
Shackling, injections.
Lesion site: finger (usually thumb)
Cheiralgia paraesthetica (work with scissors, palette).

PERIPHERAL NERVE LESIONS

Tibial nerve lesions

Causes of tibial nerve lesion

At knee level (popliteal fossa)
Baker's cyst (in rheumatoid arthritis)
Ganglion, tumour, varices
Plaster of Paris cast
Knee operations
Trauma (fracture of tibial head, knee dislocation).

In distal part of leg, ankle
Medial tarsal tunnel syndrome (flexor retinaculum compressing plantar nerve)
Fractures (distal tibia, medial malleolus, talus)
Rheumatoid disease
Phlebography and injection of varices
Tenosynovitis
Plaster of Paris pressure behind medial malleolus.

In the sole of the foot
Morton's metatarsalgia (chronic compression between third and fourth metatarsals).

Peroneal nerve lesions

Common peroneal nerve
Lesion site: knee, compression at head of fibula
Pressure palsy during anaesthesia
Plaster of Paris casts, calipers
Crossing of legs
Injuries kneeling and crouching
Knee injuries, foot inversion trauma
Extreme weight loss, with tibialis anterior syndrome
Knee operations (osteotomies, osteosyntheses, joint prostheses)
Ganglion (proximal tibiofibular joint)
Exostoses of head of fibula.

Deep peroneal nerve
Anterior tarsal tunnel syndrome (under cruciate ligaments, associated with heavy footwear).

Superficial peroneal nerve
Crossing lower legs with limbs extended
Blunt lower leg trauma.

MEMORIX NEUROLOGY

Femoral nerve lesions

With paralysis of ileopsoas muscle
Site: retroperitoneal; haematomas, possibly in psoas muscle (anticoagulation), pelvic disease (tumour, inflammation), hip replacement, aortic aneurysm, idiopathic (ischaemic).

Without paralysis of ileopsoas
Lesion site: inguinal region
Parturition, gynaecological surgery, hernia surgery, femoral angiography, lithotomy position, trauma, irradiation, hip dislocation.

Isolated saphenous nerve lesion
Lesion site: thigh
Sensory loss below knee
Compression in adductor canal, operations in medial upper thigh.

Isolated saphenous nerve lesion
Lesion site: below knee
Sensory loss lower leg and foot
Varicose vein surgery, plaster of Paris.

Isolated lesion of infrapatellar branch (plexus)
Site: insertion of sartorius
'Gonalgia paraesthetica' after knee surgery.

Sciatic nerve lesions

Lesions in buttock
Bad intramuscular injections, haematoma, surgery (hip replacement, femoral neck fracture, osteotomy), dislocation, traction in lithotomy positioning, obstetric trauma.

Lesions in pelvis
Piriformis syndrome (after trauma, sacroiliac arthropathy)
Tumour, pressure lesions.

Lesions in thigh
Fractures of femur, penetrating injuries.

Obturator nerve lesions

Lesion site: pelvis
Pelvic tumours, birth trauma, sacroiliac arthropathies, total hip replacement, pelvic fractures, obturator hernia (when pain affects the distal end of the medial thigh region: syndrome of Romberg – Howship).

Lateral cutaneus nerve of the thigh lesions

Site of lesion: retroperitoneal
Kidney transplantation, tumours and operations in iliac fossa (colon, retrocaecal appendicitis)

Site of lesion: groin
Meralgia paraesthetica (inguinal ligament, iliac fascia and fascia lata)
Plaster jacket, biopsies at pelvic rim, lymphoma.

Gluteal nerve lesions

Intramuscular injection, surgery (hip replacement), haematoma in buttock, pelvic fracture.

Pudendal nerve lesions

Space-occupying lesions, prolapse and surgery of pelvic floor (uterine prolapse).

PERIPHERAL NERVE LESIONS

Compartment syndromes

Definition
Neurogenic and myogenic paresis combined with ischaemic symptoms arising from increased pressure in fascial compartments.

Main features
Local pain with increasing pain, induration, erythema and swelling.
Late effects: contractures with electrical silence in EMG.

Causes
Fractures and their management, osteotomies; overstraining of muscles with oedema; haemorrhages, ischaemia; infusions and intra-arterial injections; plaster of Paris bandages and splinting.

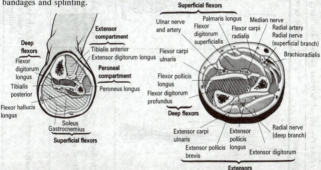

Clinically important forms

Designation	Affected compartment	Pareses	Nerve lesions	Specific causes
Tibialis anterior syndrome	Extensor compartment of leg	Tibialis anterior, extensor digitorum and extensor hallucis longus	Deep peroneal nerve	Overstrain (football, bowling), soft tissue trauma
Tibialis posterior syndrome	Deep flexor compartment of leg	Tibialis posterior, flexor digitorum and hallucis longus	Tibial nerve	Fracture and internal nailing of tibia, venous thromboses
Volkmann's ischaemic contracture	Flexor compartment of forearm	Flexor digitorum profundus and flexor pollicis longus and various other muscles	Median and ulnar, rarely radial nerve	Ischaemia (brachial artery) haemorrhage, bad injections, ulnar fractures, plaster of Paris

Differential diagnosis of important peripheral nerve lesions

(Guarantors of Brain (1976) *Aids to the Examination of the Peripheral Nervous System*, Baillière, Tindall, London.)

	Common peroneal nerve lesion	L5 root syndrome	Sciatic nerve lesion
Sensation	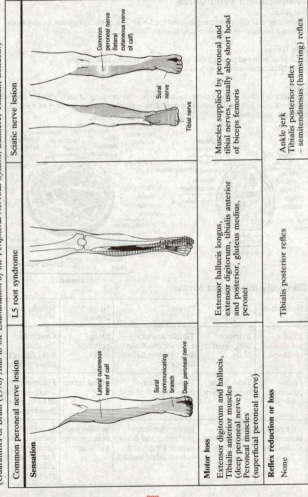		
Motor loss	Extensor digitorum and hallucis, Tibialis anterior muscles (deep peroneal nerve) Peroneal muscles (superficial peroneal nerve)	Extensor hallucis longus, extensor digitorum, tibialis anterior and posterior, gluteus medius, peronei	Muscles supplied by peroneal and tibial nerves, usually also short head of biceps femoris
Reflex reduction or loss	None	Tibialis posterior reflex	Ankle jerk Tibialis posterior reflex – semitendinosus (hamstring) reflex

PERIPHERAL NERVE LESIONS

Differential diagnosis of important peripheral nerve lesions (continued)

	Tibial nerve lesion	S1 root syndrome	Sciatic nerve lesion	Sacral plexus lesion
Sensation			(Common peroneal nerve including lateral cutaneous nerve of calf; Sural nerve; Tibial nerve)	As in sciatic nerve lesion with additional loss of back of thigh
Motor loss	Flexor digitorum, hallucis, lumbricals, abductor hallucis, tibialis posterior, gastrocnemius, soleus	Peronei, triceps surae, – gluteal muscles	All muscles supplied by common peroneal and tibial nerves	All posterior muscles supplied by common peroneal and tibialis nerves Gluteal muscles, knee flexors (positive Trendelenburg sign)
Reflex reduction or loss	Ankle jerk Posterior tibial reflex	Ankle jerk	Ankle jerk Posterior tibial reflex	Ankle jerk

Differential diagnosis of important peripheral nerve lesions (continued)

	Femoral nerve lesion	L4 root syndrome	Diabetic amyotrophy
Sensation	Medial cutaneous nerve of thigh; Saphenous nerve		No relevant sensory defect
Motor loss	Quadriceps, sartorius, pectineus muscles – ileopsoas muscle in case of high intrapelvic lesion	Quadriceps, tibialis anterior muscles – adductors	Quadriceps, adductors, hip muscles; discrete contralateral weakness
Reflex reduction or loss	Knee jerk	Knee jerk – adductor reflex	Knee jerk – adductor reflex

PERIPHERAL NERVE LESIONS

Differential diagnosis of important peripheral nerve lesions (continued)

Proximal ulnar nerve lesion	C8 root syndrome	Lower brachial plexus lesion
Sensation		
(Superficial branch, Dorsal branch, Palmar branch, Superficial branch)		Horner's syndrome
Motor loss		
Interossei, adductor pollicis, lumbricals 3 and 4, flexor digitorum profundus (ulnar half)	As for ulnar lesion plus triceps weakness	In addition extensor carpi radialis, extensor digitorum, extensor pollicis, lumbricals 1 and 2, flexor digitorum profundus (radial part) often also Horner's syndrome
Reflex reduction or loss		
Finger jerk	Finger jerk Triceps jerk	Finger jerk

Differential diagnosis of important peripheral nerve lesions (continued)

Distal median nerve lesion (carpal tunnel syndrome)	C7 root syndrome
Sensation	
Motor loss Abductor pollicis brevis, opponens pollicis, flexor pollicis brevis, lumbricals 1 and 2	In addition to thenar muscle paresis: triceps, pectoralis major (middle part), pronator teres, long finger flexors
Reflex reduction or loss None	Triceps jerk

MUSCLE DISEASES

Muscle diseases: diagnostic procedures
(Reproduced after Reichmann, H. and Mertens, H.G. (1988) Diagnostik von Myopathien. *Dtsch Aerztebl*, **85**, 2364–2368.)

Laboratory diagnosis
Serum: ESR, rheumatoid tests, immunoelectrophoresis
Acetylcholine receptor antibodies, myofibril antibodies, ENA, ANA, SMA
Lactate, pyruvate, alanine (possibly also after exertion)
CPK and isoenzyme, LDH, aldolase, electrolytes (potassium)
Urine: myoglobin, glucose, phosphate, amino acids
CSF: lactate.

Special investigations
Lactate estimation after ischaemia and on exertion (ergometer)
Electromyography (EMG), electroneurography
Muscle computerized tomography and ultrasound
Magnetic (spin echo) resonance spectroscopic measurement of creatine phosphate and ATP under aerobic and anaerobic conditions
Cardiac investigations (ECG, echocardiography, chest X-ray)

Muscle biopsy
Histology: inflammatory cells (polymyositis, vasculitis)
Scatter of fibre size, increase of lipids, dystrophin demonstration (muscular dystrophy)
Structural anomalies (congenital myopathies)
Electron microscopy: lipids, glycogen, mitochondria (mitochondrial myopathies)
Immunohistology: cellular infiltrates (lymphocytes), antigens, complement, antibodies (in myositides, collagenoses)
Biochemistry: anaerobic metabolism
Acid maltase (Pompe's disease), muscle phosphorylase (McArdle's disease), phosphofructokinase, phosphoglycerate kinase, phosphoglycerate mutase, lactate dehydrogenase
Aerobic metabolism (mitochondrial myopathies)
Pyruvate carboxylase, carnitine, respiratory chain defects
Molecular biology: genome analysis with DNA probes

Benign congenital myopathies

Definition
Congenital and usually inherited myopathy with typical histology; long-term prognosis usually good.

Clinical features
Floppy infant with muscle hypotonia, hyporeflexia and usually retarded motor development. Possibly skeletal anomalies, ophthalmoplegias.

Diagnosis
Muscle biopsy shows structural abnormalities
Central core disease: absence of NADH dehydrogenase in muscle fibre core
Multicore disease: multifocal absence of NADH dehydrogenase
Centronuclear myopathy: central location of nuclei in muscle fibres
Nemaline myopathy: inclusion (rod structures) in muscle fibres

Treatment
Prophylactic treament of infections in infants and young children; youths and adults may benefit from graded attention of remedial gymnast.

Congenital diseases of muscle

1. **Progressive muscular dystrophies**
   (a) Linked recessive inheritance
      (i) Duchenne type: infantile, poor prognosis, pelvic girdle — Defect chromosome Xp 21 – dystrophin anomaly
      (ii) Becker–Kiener type: juvenile, benign, pelvic girdle
      (iii) Emery–Dreifuss type: scapulohumeral, distal, adult, contractures
   (b) Autosomal recessive inheritance
      (i) Limb girdle type: start pelvic girdle (Leyden–Moebius), start shoulder girdle (Erb), variable — Defect chromosome 15 p
      (ii) Congenital muscular dystrophy: malignant (de Lange), benign (Batten–Turner) — Defect chromosome 6
   (c) Autosomal dominant inheritance
      (i) Facioscapulohumeral form (Landouzy–Déjerine), juvenile — Defect chromosome 4 q
      (ii) Scapulohumeral form (Erb): adult
      (iii) Scapuloperoneal form: adult
      (iv) Pelvic girdle form (Heyck–Laudahn): adult
      (v) Distal limb type: adult (Welander), infantile (Magee–Dejong)
      (vi) Ocular form (Fuchs–Kiloh–Nevin): variable
      (vii) Oculopharyngeal form (Victor): adult.

2. **Myotonias**
   (a) Autosomal dominant inheritance
      (i) Dystrophia myotonica: adult — Defect chromosome 19
      (ii) Myotonia congenita (Thomsen): infantile
      (iii) Paramyotonia congenita (Eulenburg): infantile
   (b) Autosomal recessive inheritance
      (i) Myotonia congenita (Becker): infantile
      (i) Myotonia with dwarfism (Schwartz–Jampel): infantile.

3. **Myopathic syndromes in metabolic diseases**
   (a) Enzyme defects
      (i) Glycogenoses types I–V (type II Pompe, type V McArdle, variable v. infra
      (ii) Lipid storage myopathy: infantile
      (iii) Myoglobinuria (malignant hyperthermia): juvenile
      (iv) Rhabdomyolysis (paroxysmal myoglobinuria): juvenile
      (v) Mitochondrial (Table 240)
   (b) Disorders of potassium metabolism (autosomal dominant inheritance: juvenile (Table 251)
      (i) Hypokalaemic paralysis
      (ii) Hyperkalaemic paralysis (Gamstorp)
      (iii) Normokalaemic paralysis.

MUSCLE DISEASES

Congenital diseases of muscle (continued)

4. **Congenital myopathies** (non-progressive, infantile, autosomal dominant or recessive)
   (a) Nemaline myopathy
   (b) Centro-nuclear myopathy
   (c) Central core disease.

Glycogenoses (enzyme defects of glycogen metabolism in lysosomes and muscle cytosol)
(a) **Type 2: acid maltase deficiency (1,4 glucosidase deficiency)**
   CK elevated, unstable EMG, vacuolar myopathy with glycogen storage.
   Demonstrable enzyme deficiency in muscle, fibroblasts, urine.
   (i) Pompe type in neonates: involvement of liver, heart, kidneys, CNS and PNS:
       fatal before second year
   (ii) Infantile-juvenile type (age 3–12): proximal myopathy, also respiratory muscles, death usually before age 20
   (iii) Adult type (after age 20): focal proximal myopathy with selective hypertrophy,
       trunk and respiratory muscles also involved, sleep disorders common
   Attempt treatment with high protein, low carbohydrate diet.
(b) **Other types**
   (i) Type 3: Forbes' disease: debranching enzyme deficiency (amylo-1,6 glucosidase deficiency; children with proximal myopathy and hepatomegaly
   (ii) Type 4: Branching enzyme deficiency (amylo-1,4-1,6 transglucosidase deficiency) congenital or neonates: liver cirrhosis, very poor prognosis
   (iii) Type 5: **McArdle's disease (muscle phosphorylase deficiency):** mostly prepubertal, commoner in boys, exertion-related myalgia, weakness, stiffness, oedema with myoglobinuria
   (iv) Type 7: Phospho-fructokinase deficiency: men, juveniles, related to exertion, erythrocytes involved.

Mitochondrial myopathies

(Reproduced after Reichmann, H. (1988) *Dtsch Med Wschr*, **113**, 196; Jerusalem, F. and Ziers, S. (1991) *Muskelerkrankungen*, Thieme, Stuttgart; Di Mauro, S. *et al.* (1985) *Annals of Neurology*, **17**, 521–538.)

Definition
Myopathy based on mitochondrial enzyme defect, mostly of mitochondrial or autosomal recessive inheritance, which can affect:
1. Substrate transport in mitochondria, e.g. carnitine-palmityl transferase.
2. Mitochondrial substrate utilization, e.g. pyruvate dehydrogenase.
3. Mitochondrial respiratory chain, e.g. enzyme complexes, coenzyme Q.
4. Oxidative phosphorylation, e.g. ATPase, Luft's syndrome.

Clinical features
Weakness and pain of musculature, especially on sustained exertion; chronic progressive external ophthalmoplegia (CPEO), inadequate respiration, cardiomyopathy.

Laboratory tests
Raised blood lactate (especially after exertion and ischaemia testing), occasionally raised CK, pyruvate, alanine, glycosuria, amino aciduria, phosphaturia with cytochrome oxidase deficiency.

Muscle biopsy diagnostic features
On microscopy: ragged red fibres; on electron microscopy: mitochondrial aggregates and alterations, possibly also accumulation of glycogen and lipid; biochemical analysis of mitochondria for enzyme defects.

Variants

	Enzyme defect	Age of onset	Clinical features	Electron microscopy	Laboratory tests	Prognosis	Treatment
Pyruvate metabolism	Pyruvate dehydrogenase	Baby	Floppy infant	Lipid accumulation	Lactate pyruvate alanine	Lethal	None
Lipid metabolism	Carnitine deficiency	Children Adults	Paresis Hepatic encephalopathy	Lipid accumulation	Carnitine (in muscle) occasionally ketoacidosis	Grave if systematized, otherwise good	Acute: glucose iv, then oral carnitine
	Carnitine-palmitoyl transferase deficiency	Children	Myalgia Exertional myoglobinuria	Often unremarkable	Lactate, CK, myoglobinuria	Good	Diet low fat and high carbohydrate; avoid exertion
Respiratory chain	Complex 1 deficiency	Children	Paresis on prolonged exertion	Ragged red fibres	Lactate	Variable	Vitamin C and K (?)
	Complex II–III defect	Children	Encephalomyopathy	–	–	–	
	Cytochrome C oxidase deficiency	Baby	Floppy infant	–	–	Often fatal, rarely benign	

MUSCLE DISEASES

Malignant hyperthermia

A genetic predisposition to develop malignant hyperpyrexia from trigger drugs (inhalational anaesthetics and depolarizing muscle relaxants): compare the neuroleptic malignant syndrome
Incidence 1 in 75 000 general anaesthetics in adults (commoner in children).

Clinical features
Tachycardia with abnormal rhythms, tachypnoea, muscular rigidity (jaw muscles), labile blood pressure: as the condition progresses metabolic acidosis with electrolyte disorders, cyanosis, hyperthermia, rhabdomyolysis with myoglobinuria. Danger of renal and left ventricular failure, coagulopathy. Mortality 10–30%.

Triggering agents
Halothane, suxamethonium – rarely other anaesthetic agents (also neuroleptic malignant syndrome from fluphenazine etc).

Hints of predisposition
Earlier anaesthetic mishaps, family history of muscle diseases, myalgia with fever, dark urine after anaesthesia, or spontaneous, unexplained deaths in the family.
Raised phosphocreatine-kinase (in about 70% prior to drug exposure), skeletal deformities (scoliosis, abnormal feet), flaccid connective tissue with propensity to hernias.

Diagnostic tests
Creatine kinase, TRH test, lipid electrophoresis
Muscle ischaemia test with lactate and ammonium estimation
EMG
Muscle biopsy under local anaesthesia for histology, histochemistry and *in vitro* study of halothane-induced contracture.

Management
Withdrawal of potential trigger substances
Infusion of dantrolene sodium
Ventilation and iv injection of sodium bicarbonate according to degree of acidosis
Cooling
Diuretics
If further anaesthesia is required: neuroleptanalgesia, nitrous oxide, barbiturates, benzodiazepines, pancuronium.

Prophylaxis
Registration of patients at risk of malignant hyperpyrexia
If possible use local anaesthesia, otherwise use prophylactic dantrolene 30 min before anaesthesia
Anaesthetize with barbiturates, opiates, benzodiazepines, nitrous oxide, pancuronium.

Muscular dystrophies: genetics and course

	Age of onset (years)	Years of life expectancy	Clinical features
X chromosome (recessive) inheritance (all males)			
Duchenne type	1–3	20–30	Pelvic girdle, pseudohypertrophy, Gower's sign, cardiomyopathy, demonstration of dystrophin, genetic studies
Becker–Kiener type	6–20	30–60	
Emery–Dreifuss type	5–15	50–60	
McLeod type	No clinical manifestation		Scapulohumeral distal, contractures, heart rhythm disorders, EMG abnormalities, acanthocytosis (erythrocytes)
Autosomal recessive inheritance (M and F)			
Limb girdle type	2–50	60–70	Mostly scapulohumeral at first, then descending
congenital muscular dystrophy	At birth	Variable	Floppy infant, combination with arthrogryphosis multiplex
Autosomal dominant inheritance (M and F)			
Facioscapulohumeral muscular dystrophy (Landouzy–Dejerine)	10–20	Normal	Starts in face, possibly with pains
Scapuloperoneal muscular dystrophy	20–40	Normal	Shoulder girdle and below knees, upper arms
Distal limb type: adult	40–60	Normal	Distal limb muscles, spreading proximally
: infantile	2–15	Normal	
Ocular muscular dystrophy	Variable	Normal	Chronic progressive external ophthalmoplegia
Oculopharyngeal muscular dystrophy	40–60	Normal	Eye movements first, then swallowing
Myotonia: autosomal dominant inheritance			
Myotonia dystrophica (Curschmann–Steiner)	15–30	50–60	Myotonia (tongue, thenar), myopathic facies, distal limb muscles, cardiac conduction block, cataracts, nerve deafness, frontal baldness, endocrine disorders, skeletal deformities

MUSCLE DISEASES

Mitochondrial multisystem disorders (myo-encephalopathies) from point mutations of mitochondrial DNA

(Reproduced after Di Mauro, A. *et al.* (1985) Mitochondrial myopathies. *Annals of Neurology*, **17**, 521–538.)

LHON (Leber's hereditary optic neuropathy)

Enzyme defect: complex I deficiency detectable in muscle
Clinical features: progressive blindness from optic atrophy; maternal inheritance
Age of onset: 10th–30th year
Diagnostic tests: CK, LDH, lactate in serum. Molecular biology. Muscle biopsy with biochemical assessment

MELAS (myoencephalopathy with lactic acidosis and strokes)

Enzyme defect: in respiratory chain (cytochrome-C-oxidase, succinate-cytochrome-C-reductase)
Clinical features: epilepsy (focal and/or generalized), migrainous headaches, episodic paralyses, muscle hypotonia, dementia, episodic vomiting, stroke episodes with hemianopia, hemiparesis, growth retardation
Age of onset: newborn, young children. Familial prevalence 30–40%
Diagnostic tests: CK, GOT, LDH, lactate in serum. Basal ganglia calcification in CT, EMG, EEG Muscle biopsy including biochemistry. Ischaemia test. Molecular biology

MERRF (myoclonus epilepsy and ragged red fibres)

Enzyme defect: succinate-cytochrome-C-reductase
Clinical features: myoclonus, ataxia, generalized epilepsy, dementia, optic atrophy, pareses, growth retardation, deafness
Age of onset: 10th–20th year. Familial prevalence 60–70%, maternal inheritance
Diagnostic tests: muscle Gomori trichrome stain (ragged red fibres), ischaemia test, CK, GOT, LDH. Molecular biology

NARP (neuropathy, ataxia and retinitis pigmentosa)

Enzyme defect: succinate-cytochrome-C-reductase
Clinical features: retinitis pigmentosa, developmental retardation, ataxia, epilepsy, dementia, proximal neurogenic muscle weakness, growth retardation, sensory neuropathy
Age of onset: childhood, maternal inheritance
Diagnostic tests: muscle biopsy, molecular biology

MEMORIX NEUROLOGY

Mitochondrial multisystem disorders (myo-encephalopathies) from point mutations of mitochondrial DNA (Continued)

(Reproduced after Di Mauro, A. et al. (1985) Mitochondrial myopathies. *Annals of Neurology*, **17**, 521–538.)

PEO (progressive external ophthalmoplegia and KSS (Kearns–Sayre syndrome)

Enzyme defect:	cytochrome-aa3-oxidase, cytochrome-C-oxidase
Clinical features:	myopathy of external eye muscles (PEO), in KSS also retinitis, ataxia, growth retardation, cardiac conduction defects as part of cardiomyopathy, myopathy, deafness, epilepsy, dementia
Age of onset:	10th–20th year; sporadic appearance. PEO may show autosomal dominant inheritance
Diagnostic tests:	raised CSF protein (in 70%); muscle biochemistry, ischaemia test. CK, GOT, LDH. EMG, ECG, etc. Molecular biology
Treatment:	coenzyme Q 10, occasionally cardiac pacemaker.

Symptoms and signs	KSS	MERRF	MELAS
Ophthalmoplegia	+	−	−
Retinal degeneration	+	−	−
Heart block	+	−	−
Myoclonias	−	+	−
Ataxia	±	+	+
Muscle weakness	+	+	+
Cerebral attacks	−	+	+
Episodic vomiting	−	−	+
Cortical blindness	−	−	+
Hemipareses	−	−	+
Other neurological defects	±	±	±
High blood lactate	+	+	+
Ragged red fibres	+	+	+

MUSCLE DISEASES

Myopathies: metabolic function tests
(Reproduced after Jerusalem, F. and Zierz, S. *Muskelerkrankungen*, published by Thieme, Stuttgart, 1991.)

Ischaemia test

1. Bodily rest for 1 h.
2. Basal values from venous sample from untested and unconstricted arm.
3. Blood pressure cuff on tested arm inflated to 30 mmHg above systolic RR reading.
4. Patient forcibly compresses a rubber ball 60 times in 1 min with (tested) hand.
5. Release blood pressure cuff.
6. Blood samples after 1, 3, 5 and 10 min from cubital vein of tested arm.
7. Instant deproteination of samples by ice-cold perchloric acid.
8. Rapid estimation of lactate, pyruvate and ammonium.

Normal ranges of increase (absolute values)
Lactate: 3.5 ± 1.1 mmol/l (2.4–5.9)
Pyruvate: 131 ± 43 µmol/l (63–197)
Ammonium: 105 ± 39 µmol/l (28–190)

Interpretation	
No increase of lactate Normal increase of ammonium	Defect of glycolysis or glycogenolysis
No increase of ammonium Normal increase of lactate	Myoadenylate deaminase deficiency
No or reduced increase of both lactate and ammonium	Paresis or failure to comply
Normal increase of enzymes	Normal result (but does not exclude enzyme defect)

Ergometer test

1. Rest for 30 min.
2. Venous blood test from unconstricted arm (for basal levels).
3. Bicycle ergometer (load 30 Watt) for 15 min.
4. Blood tests every 5 min during exertion.
5. Last blood test 15 min after end of exertion.
6. Instant deproteination of samples by ice-cold perchloric acid.
7. Rapid estimation of lactate and pyruvate.
8. Determination of lactate/pyruvate quotient.

Normal ranges of increase (absolute values) – see above for ischaemia test

Interpretation	
Little or no increase on exertion	Normal result (false negatives in up to 20%)
Pathological increase on exertion, with or without pathological basal values	Mitochondrial myopathy, pyruvate dehydrogenase deficiency, other severe myopathies

MEMORIX NEUROLOGY

Causes of myoglobinuria

(Reproduced after Brass, L. and Stys, P. *Handbook of Neurological Lists*, published by Churchill Livingstone, New York, 1991.)

Hereditary
- McArdle's disease (muscle phosphorylase deficiency)
- Phospho-fructokinase deficiencey
- Carnitine-palmityl-transferase deficiency
- Malignant hyperpyrexia.

Acquired
- Muscular overload (sport, tibialis anterior syndrome, epileptic fits, tetanus, dystonias, alcoholic delirium, catatonia)

- Trauma, infection, electric shock, burns, air embolism, prolonged coma, heat stroke, hypothermia, barotrauma, toxic shock syndrome, sepsis

- Myopathies (polymyositis, dermatomyositis, alcoholic myopathy, leptospirosis)

- Toxic (anaesthesia, barbiturates, carbon monoxide, succinyl choline, amphotericin B, heroin, neuroleptics (neuroleptic malignant syndrome), food poisoning, snake bite, alcohol)

- Metabolic (diabetic ketoacidosis, hypokalaemia, hypophosphataemia).

Disorders of electrical membrane stability: ion channel disorders

Myotonias and periodic paralyses (g_{Cl}, g_{Na}, g_K indicate sarcolemmal permeability for Cl^-, Na^+, K^+: ↑ increased, ↓ reduced)

Disease (original author)	Inheritance	Membrane defect
Myotonia congenita (Thomsen)	Dominant	g_{Na} ↓
Recessive generalized myotonia (Becker)	Recessive	g_{Cl} ↓
Dystrophia myotonica (Steinert)	Dominant	g_{Cl} ↓ ?, g_{Na} ↑ ?
Paramyotonia congenita (Eulenburg)	Dominant	g_{Na} ↑
Familial hyperkalaemic periodic paralysis	Dominant	g_{Na} ↑
Fanilial hypokalaemic paralysis (Westphal)	Dominant	g_{Na}/g_K ↑
Secondary periodic paralyses	Sporadic	?

MUSCLE DISEASES

Grading of myasthenia gravis

(Reproduced after Osserman, K.E. and Genkins, G. (1971) Studies in myasthenia gravis. *Mount Sinai Journal of Medicine*, **38**, 497–537.)

I	Localized non-progressive form of myasthenia; excellent prognosis (e.g. ocular myasthenia)
IIa	Slow onset generalized myasthenia, frequently ocular at first, spreading to affect more than one group of striated muscle, sparing of respiratory muscles. Usually amenable to drug treatment. Fairly good prognosis
IIb	Moderate generalized form with involvement of bulbar muscles prognosis fair
III	Rapid and fulminating onset of generalized myasthenia with early respiratory involvement. Progression usually complete by 6 months. Poor response to medication and poor prognosis
IV	Late severe myasthenia which evolves within 2 years of onset in groups I and II and then behaves clinically like group III
V	Myasthenia with localized muscular atrophy: most patients present as in group II and develop muscular atrophy within 6 months of onset. Prognosis is variable and depends on other clinical features

Motor (neuromuscular) end-plate

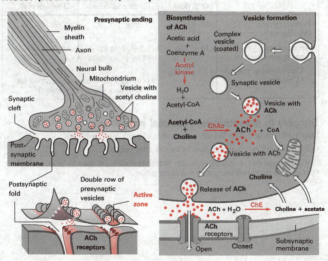

Tensilon test

Preparation Aspirate 1 ml = 10 mg Tensilon (edrophonium hydrochloride) into a syringe.
Aspirate atropine 2 mg into a second syringe as possible antidote.

Test Intravenous injection of 0.2 ml: if tolerated, inject the remaining 0.8 ml after 30 s interval.

In case of muscarinic side-effects, such as bradycardia, immediately inject the atropine.

Interpretation Depends on effect on existing clinical symptoms and signs (ptosis, diplopia, ability to maintain posture of elevated limbs or head; possibility of assessment by EMG with repetitive stimulation of nerve). Assessment of any effect 20–30 s after injection – may last up to 10 min.

(Tensilon may cause some twitching of normal and particularly of denervated muscles.)

Prostigmine may serve as an alternative and longer-lasting test substance.

Myasthenia treatment: anticholinesterases (doses for adults)

	Oral dose	Parenteral dose	Dose interval
Pyridostigmine (Mestinon)	60–180 mg	3–6 mg	4–6 h
Neostigmine (Prostigmine)	15–30 mg	0.5–1.0 mg im or by iv injection	4 h
Edrophonium chloride (Tensilon)		1–10 mg by intravenous injection for testing only (very short acting)	

Surgery in myasthenia: practical procedures

Stop azathioprine 2 days before, restart, second week after operation.

Corticosteroids: no change in dose before or after operation.

Anticholinesterases: continue up to day before operation, re-start by mouth 6 h after operation; if necessary use parenteral neostigmine.

MUSCLE DISEASES

Differentiation of myasthenic from cholinergic crisis

	Myasthenic crisis	Cholinergic crisis
Eye	Pupil medium or dilated	Pupil constricted Accommodation failure (distant look)
Breathing	Respiration poor from muscle paresis	Respiration poor from muscle paresis, bronchial constriction and increased bronchial secretions
Heart	Tachycardia	Bradycardia
Abdomen	Possibly urge to defaecate	Abdominal cramps, diarrhoea
Muscles	Flaccid paresis	Flaccid paresis with fasciculations and calf cramps
Skin	Pale, possibly cold	Erythematous, warm
Procedure and Treatment	Tensilon test positive (stronger) Prostigmine 0.5 mg iv injection then Mestinon 24 mg in 500 ml glucose iv infusion; if required suction, intubation, ventilation	Tensilon test negative (weaker, ISQ) Atropine 2 mg iv injection, if required suction, intubation, ventilation

Note: possibility of mixed crisis – if so initiate ventilation, stop anticholinesterases, consider use of corticosteroids and/or plasmapheresis

Myasthenia: medications to be avoided and alternatives

(Modified from Hartmann, A. *et al.* (1987) Thymektomie Dei Myasthenia gravis. *Aktuel Neurol*, **14**, 26–27.)

Prohibited medications	Alternative medications
Antibiotics Aminoglycosides Polymyxin Tetracycline Lincomycin Clindomycin High-dose penicillin Sulphonamides	Cephalosporin Erythromycin Chloramphenicol Nitrofurantoin Penicillin (low dose) Nalidixic acid Tuberculo-statics (INH, rifampicin)
Anticonvulsants Phenytoin Barbiturates Benzodiazepines (high dose)	Carbamazepine Primidone Sodium valproate
Psychotropic drugs Neuroleptics Lithium Benzodiazepines (high dose) Amitriptyline	Thioridazine Benzodiazepines (low dose) Promethazine Chlorpromazine
Endocrine preparations ACTH Corticosteroids Oral contraceptives Oxytocin Thyroid hormones	Corticosteroids permissible under strict clinical control
Cardiovascular preparations Anti-arrhythmics (quinidine, lignocaine, procainamide) Beta-blockers Ganglion blocking agents Benethiazide Guanethidine	Digitalis Reserpine Methyl DOPA Spironolactone Triamterene
Analgesics, antirheumatics and anti-inflammatory agents	
Morphine derivatives Quinine Chloroquine d-penicillamine Antimalarials	Acetylsalicylic acid Phenylbutazone Indomethacin Pentazocine Gold

Muscle relaxants may only be used under intensive care monitoring conditions

MULTIFOCAL NEUROLOGICAL DISORDERS

Dyskalaemic periodic paralyses

	Hypokalaemic periodic paralysis	Hyperkalaemic periodic paralysis (adynamia hereditaria episodica of Gamsdorp)
Age of onset	10th–20th year	Before 10th year
Sex	M:F = 3:1	M = F
Heredity	Autosomal dominant, incomplete penetrance	Autosomal dominant
Attack frequency	Every 2–3 months	Several per day, up to weekly
Attack duration	8 h up to 4 days	Minutes up to 4 h
Start	Often in sleep	During day, especially mornings
Clinical signs	Generalized paralysis sparing facial muscles	Mild paresis, often only partial (legs)
Potassium during attack	Reduced (down to 1.8 mmol/l)	Raised (up to 7.3 mmol/l), or normal
Aldosterone during attack	Raised	Reduced
Pathogenesis	Overcompensation for raised Na flow	Disordered K reabsorption
Provoked by	Carbohydrate supply, insulin, night sleep, Na supply	K supply, rest after exertion, alcohol
Treatment in attack	KCl 2–10 g by mouth, effervescent potassium tablets	Sweets, glucose, calcium gluconate iv, metered salbutamol aerosol
Interval treatment	Low muscular exertion, low carbohydrate diet, acetazolamide, diclofenac, spironolactone	Low muscular exertion, hydrochlorothiazide, acetazolamide
Specific variants	Hypokalaemic paralysis with thyrotoxicosis	Normokalaemic paralysis, occurs in myotonia congenita
Symptomatic occurence in	Diarrhoea, vomiting, Conn's syndrome, renal tubular acidosis; drug-related (steroids, relaxants, amphotericin B, carbenoxolone, frusemide and other diuretics)	Addison's disease, chronic renal failure, myoglobinuria, drugs (spironolactone, long-term heparin)

Multifocal neurological disorders
Paraneoplastic neurological disorders

(Reproduced after Berlit, P. (1989) Paraneoplastische Syndrome. *Zentralbl Neurol.*, **252**, 3–6.)

	Occurs with	Autoantibody
Brain		
Encephalomyelitis		
Limbic encephalitis	Small cell bronchial carcinoma,	Myelin protein IgG
Bulbar encephalitis	rarely breast, ovarian, colonic	Purkinje cell IgG
Spinocerebellar degeneration	carcinomas	Neuronal IgG
Myoclonus-opsoclonus syndrome		
Progressive multifocal leucoencephalopathy	Lymphomas, leukaemias	–
Isolated CNS angiitis	Hodgkin's disease	–
Subacute cerebellar degeneration	Ovarian and breast carcinoma	Purkinje cell IgG
Spinal cord		
Subacute necrotizing myelopathy	Small cell bronchial carcinoma	IgG
Motor neuron disease	Lymphomas, bronchial, breast, gastrointestinal tract carcinomas	–
Stiff man syndrome	Bronchial carcinoma, lymphoma, breast carcinoma, thymoma	IgG
Peripheral nerve		
Subacute sensory neuropathy (often concurrent encephalomyelitis)	Small cell bronchial carcinoma	Antineuronal Ig
Paraproteinaemic polyneuropathy	Plasmacytoma, lymphoma	Monoclonal Ig
Sensory-motor polyneuropathy	Bronchial carcinoma	Ig, MAG
Guillain–Barré syndrome	Lymphoma	IgG
Neuromuscular system		
Eaton Lambert syndrome	Small cell bronchial carcinoma	Calcium channel IgG
Myasthenia gravis	Thymoma	Striated muscle IgG
Muscle		
Polymyositis, dermatomyositis	Breast, bronchial, gastrointestinal tract, uterine, ovarian carcinoma	Muscle IgG

MEMORIX NEUROLOGY

Neurological features of endocrine disorders

(Reproduced after Dale, A. (1972) Neurological problems in endocrine diseases. *Medical Clinics of North America*, 56, 1029–1039.)

Parathyroid

Hyperparathyroidism
Psychological symptoms (fatigue, confusion, personality change, anxiety)
Muscular weakness

Hypoparathyroidism
Tetany
Epileptic fits
Psychological symptoms (confusion, restlessness, hallucinations)
Chorea
Basal ganglia calcification

Thyroid

Hyperthyroidism
Myopathy
Myasthenia gravis
Hypokalaemic periodic paralysis
Exophthalmus (ophthalmopathy)
Tremor, restlessness, tension
Polyneuropathy (rarely)

Hypothyroidism
Carpal tunnel syndrome
Myopathy
Polyneuropathy
Cerebellar degeneration
Disordered consciousness up to coma

Adrenal cortex

Addison's disease
Apathy, fatiguability, anxiety
Hyperkalaemic paralysis
Heat cramps

Cushing's disease
Sleep disorders, restlessness, psychotic symptoms, myopathy

Primary aldosteronism
Hypokalaemic paralysis

Adrenal medulla

Phaeochromocytoma
Headache in hypertensive crises
Intracerebral haemorrhage

Pancreas

Diabetes mellitus
Diabetic coma
Polyneuropathy with autonomic involvement
Diabetic amyotrophy
Cranial nerve mononeuropathy (III nerve)

Hyperinsulinism (islet cell tumour)
Hypoglycaemic coma
Symptomatic fits
Focal neurological signs in hypoglycaemia
Neuronal damage

Pituitary, hypothalamus

Local pressure effects
Bitemporal hemianopia
Cranial nerve palsies (superior orbital fissure and cavernous sinus syndromes)
Obstructive hydrocephalus

Endocrine features of hypersecreting pituitary tumours

Endocrine features of hypothalamic dysfunction
Diabetes insipidus
Syndrome of inappropriate antidiuretic hormone secretion (SIADH)

MULTIFOCAL NEUROLOGICAL DISORDERS

Multiple sclerosis: classification

A **Definite multiple sclerosis**
Two relapses or progression over the course of 1 year

+

At least two disseminated symptoms and signs
(allowing for neurophysiological findings)

+

Typical CSF changes
(intrathecal IgG production, oligoclonal bands, mild mononuclear pleocytosis)

+

Multifocal white matter lesions demonstrated in MRI.

B **Probable multiple sclerosis**
At least two of the criteria listed above under A have been satisfied.

C **Possible multiple sclerosis**
Symptoms and signs which could indicate multiple sclerosis, but at time in question no evidence of relapses in time, or of multiplicicty of lesions favouring diagnosis, e.g. isolated retrobulbar neuritis.

Impairment (Kurtzke) scale in multiple sclerosis

(Reproduced after Kurtzke, J.F. (1963) Rating neurological impairment in multiple sclerosis. *Neurology (Minneap)*, **33**, 1444–1452.)

0 Normal findings

1 No disability, minimal signs

2 Minimal disability in one functional system (e.g. slight spasticity or paresis)

3 Moderate disability in one functional system, or mild disability in 3 or 4 systems

4 Disability which impairs but does not prohibit normal job and life style

5 Partial inability to work, maximal walking distance without aid 200 m

6 Walking limited to 100 m with support from sticks, props

7 Wheel-chair bound patient who can get in and out of, and move chair, without help

8 Bed or chair-bound but retains effective use of upper limbs

9 Helpless bed-ridden patient

10 Death from multiple sclerosis.

Multiple sclerosis – CAMBS scale
(Mumford, C. and Compston, A. (1993) Rating scale for multiple sclerosis. *Journal of Neurology*, **240**, 209–215.)

Disability and impairment
- unknown
1. Patient is fully independent.
2. Patient with only one symptom of: mild fatigue, visual blurring (can read), minor sensory symptoms or sphincter disturbance, altered arm function, or mild difficulty walking.
3. Patient with one or more of: frequency and continence problems, definite visual disorder (cannot read), inability to use one or both arms, marked pain or dysaesthesiae, requires bilateral supports to walk, clear intellectual impairment.
4. Wheel-chair-bound patient, or other major disability restricting daily activities.
5. Bed-ridden, or otherwise entirely care dependent.

Relapse
- unknown
1. Quiescent, or non-relapsing course.
2. Subjectively worse but improving or objectively unchanged.
3. Subjectively worse; worse than base-line and deteriorating.
4. Worse as result of established relapse.
5. Major deterioration necessitating hospital admission and increased dependency.

Progression
- no knowledge of illness up to present time
1. Apart from recent changes clinically unaltered for last year.
2. Minor deterioration in past year.
3. Significant disability in past year.
4. Rapid increase in disability in past year.
5. Devastating progression in past year, i.e. malignant form of disease.

Handicap
Ask patient to mark the line below to score for handicap on scale 1 to 5: 'How severely does your condition affect your ability to perform a normal role in life? Level 1 would indicate no effect on life, occupation, ability to support family. Level 5 means rendered completely incapable of any useful role in life, totally prevents normal social role, job, family life. Make mark on any digit on the line'.

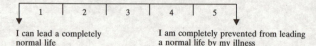

I can lead a completely normal life   I am completely prevented from leading a normal life by my illness

Multiple sclerosis: typical features

(Reproduced after Frick, E. *Multiple Sklerose*, published by VCH, Weinheim, 1987.)

Typical clinical symptoms and signs	Frequency (%)	(As presenting symptom or sign)
Sensory disorders	86	(42)
Spasticity, pyramidal tract signs	85	(29)
Central pareses	85	(45)
Cerebellar/brain stem features	79	(24)
Retrobulbar neuritis	62	(33)
Sphincter disorders	61	(9)
Altered higher mental functions	39	(4)
Eye muscle weakness	36	(14)
Other cranial nerve defects	30	(10)
Typical CSF abnormalities		
Mononuclear pleocytosis up to 50 cells/mm^3	60	
Total protein normal or slightly raised up to 100 mg%	70	
Intrathecal IgG production	80	
Oligoclonal bands detectable	≥90	
Typical neurophysiological features		
Visual evoked potentials (VEP) Prolonged latency Flattened potentials	70	
Auditory evoked potentials (AEP) Interpeak latencies lengthened Amplitude reduction peak V	70	
Somatosensory evoked potentials (SSEP) Prolonged latencies Flattening of potentials	60	
Motor evoked potentials (MEP) Central motor conduction times lengthened Amplitude reduction	70	
Typical neuroradiological findings		
CT evidence of demyelination	50	
MRI evidence of demyelination	≥90	

Matthews, W.B. (ed.) (1991) McAlpine's Multiple Sclerosis, 2nd edn, Churchill Livingstone, Edinburgh

Phacomatoses

	Age of manifestation	Inheritance	Manifestations Oculocutaneous	Manifestations Neurological	Main features
Neurofibromatosis (von Recklinghausen)	Adults	Autosomal dominant, defect chromosome 17	Subcutaneous neurofibromata, café-au-lait patches, iris anomalies, hamartoma	Cerebral, spinal and peripheral tumours (meningioma, schwannoma, glioma, neurofibroma)	Signs of space occupation, epilepsy, dementia, scoliosis
Bilateral acoustic neurofibromatosis	10–30 years	Autosomal dominant, defect chromosome 22	Neurofibromata	Bilateral acoustic schwannoma, glioma, meningioma	Deafness
Tuberous sclerosis (Bourneville)	1–3 years	Autosomal dominant	Adenoma sebaceum (face), hypopigmented patches, retinal tumours	Periventricular gliosis and calcification	Epilepsy (infantile spasms), mental retardation
Encephalofacial angiomatosis Sturge–Weber	Children or young adults	Sporadic	Capillary naevus (first and second trigeminal division), venous skin angioma, buphthalmus, glaucoma	Ipsilateral (calcified) angioma, mostly parieto-occipital with hemiatrophy	Epilepsy, focal neurological signs, mental retardation
Cerebelloretinal angiomatosis von Hippel–Lindau	Young adults	Autosomal dominant	Haemangioblastoma of retina, also kidney, pancreas	Cerebellar haemangioblastoma	Ataxia, raised intracranial pressure
Ataxia-telangiectasia Louis–Bar	Children	Autosomal recessive	Cutaneous and conjunctival telangiectasia	Cerebellar atrophy	Ataxia, retardation, infections (if IgA deficiency)
Basal cell naevoid syndrome Gorlin–Goltz	Young adults	Not uniform	Multiple basal cell lesions, jaw cysts	Ventricular dilatation falx and tentorial calcification	Epileptic fits
Racemose retinocerebral angiomatosis Wyburn–Mason	Children	Not uniform	Unilateral retinal vascular malformation, possibly also facial skin	Brain stem vascular malformation	Spastic weakness

MULTIFOCAL NEUROLOGICAL DISORDERS

The porphyrias

Erythropoietic forms
(autosomal recessive inheritance)
- Erythropoietic porphyria
- erythropoietic coproporphyria.

Erythropoietic protoporphyria
(autosomal dominant inheritance)

Hepatic prophyria
(autosomal dominant inheritance)
- Acute intermittent porphyria
- Porphyria variegata
- Hereditary coproporphyria.

Symptomatic porphyrias
- Porphyria cutanea tarda
- Toxic aetiology
- Liver diseases.

Clinical suspicion of porphyria when there is:
- Coincidence of abdominal colics with neuropsychiatric symptoms
- Polyneuropathy (mainly motor and proximal).

Test urine for:
- δ-amino-laevulinic acid
- Porphobilinogen.

Prohibited medications in porphyria and permissible alternatives

Prohibited	Permissible
Sedatives, tranquillizers	
Barbiturates	Chloral hydrate
Chlordiazepoxide	Chlorpromazine
Diazepam, oxazepam	
Meprobamate	
Anticonvulsants	
Ethosuximide	
Clonazepam, sodium valproate	
Phenytoin, primidone	
Anticoagulants	Aspirin
Centrally acting drugs	
Imipramine, nikethamide	Droperidol
Metoclopramide	Methadone (physeptone)
Methyl-dopa	Chlorpromazine, promethazine
Chemotherapeutics and antibiotics	
Sulphonamides	Gentamicin
Nalidixic acid, griseofulvin	Cephalosporin
Nitrofurantoin	Penicillin
Antihelmintics	
Analgesics, anti-inflammatory and antirheumatic agents	
Chloroquine	Aspirin
Diclofenac	Morphine (and derivatives)
Pentazocine	
Phenylbutazone	
Phenazone	
Anaesthetic agents	
Halothane, lignocaine, enflurane	Ether, fentanyl
	Suxamethonium, prilocaine
	Bupivacaine
Hormones	
Progestogens, oestrogens	Prednisolone
Progesterone	Dexamethasone
Oral contraceptives	
Others	
Theophylline, phenoxybenzamine	Digitalis
Spironolactone, pyrimethamine	Propanolol, reserpine
Tolbutamide	Atropine
Hydralazine	Cimetidine
Ergotamine	Guanethidine
Clonidine	

For further information refer to the British National Formulary

Alcoholism: disorders of the nervous system and muscle

Occasional fits
Single or serial grand mal attacks, no focal features, no specific EEG changes
No indication for long-term anticonvulsant treatment (after 'drying out').

Features of alcoholism prior to stage of delirium
Rest tremor, increased sweating, tachycardia, motor restlessness, anxiety, flushing of face (hours after alcohol withdrawn).

Delirium tremens
Disorientation, visual blocking, visual hallucinations, suggestibility, psychomotor restlessness with tension and anxiety, tachycardia, tachypnoea, hyperhidrosis, fluctuating blood pressure, hyperthermia, tremor (1–2 days after alcohol withdrawal).

Alcoholic hallucinosis
Auditory hallucinations with restlessness and anxiety. No disorder of alertness, no autonomic symptoms, no disorientation (after alcoholic over-indulgence).

Cerebellar degeneration
Ataxia of stance and gait. Abnormal heel-knee-shin test. Possibly abnormality of eye movements (in chronic alcoholism – reversible in early stages with abstinence).

Wernicke's encephalopathy
Directional nystagmus, gaze palsies, external ocular muscle palsies (VI nerve), pupillary abnormalities, internuclear ophthalmoplegia, trunk and limb ataxia, psychological defects (disorientation, restlessness, apathy, somnolence) – caused by vitamin B_1 deficiency from dietary failings.

Korsakoff's psychosis
Disorientation in time and place, failure of registration and short-term memory, confabulation – association with, or consequence of, Wernicke's encephalopathy.

Corpus callosum degeneration (Marchiafava – Bignami syndrome)
Failure of higher mental functions, primitive reflexes, disorders of consciousness, gait disorders, dysarthria (excessive red wine consumption).

Central pontine myelinolysis
Disordered consciousness, pyramidal tract signs, eye movement disorders; may progress to locked-in syndrome (associated with over-rapid correction, or over-correction of hyponatraemia).

Polyneuropathy
Symmetrical distal and mainly sensory variety with liability to pressure palsies, occasionally spontaneous pain and hyperpathia (in chronic alcohol abusers).

Tobacco-alcohol amblyopia
Deterioration of vision, central scotomata, optic disc pallor (in vitamin B and especially vitamin B_{12} deficiencies).

Acute myopathy
Painful swelling and weakness of limb and trunk muscles from rhabdomyolysis, with hyperkalaemia and myoglobinuria – risk of renal failure (after alcoholic excesses).

Chronic myopathy
Weakness and atrophy of pelvic and shoulder girdle muscles without pain (in chronic alcohol abuse).

Hypokalaemic myopathy
Proximal limb weakness without pain (with hypokalaemia, e.g. diarrhoea and vomiting).

MULTIFOCAL NEUROLOGICAL DISORDERS

Alcohol withdrawal: principles of management
Sedation with oral chlormethiazole but patient must remain arousable at all times
Vitamin B_1 100 mg daily
Correction of hypokalaemia and potassium supplementation
Ample fluid intake
Neuroleptics only in combination with tranquillizers (epileptic threshold), avoid anticonvulsants if possible – then withdraw alcohol
In case of hyponatraemia correct slowly by 1 mmol/l per hour to slightly subnormal levels, secondary to risk of central pontine myelinolysis
In presence of high creatine kinase levels beware of renal failure and consider resorting to plasmapheresis.

Neurological causes of disorders of swallowing
(Modified from Hörmann, M. *et al.* (1988) Oropharyngeal Dysphagie bei neuromuskulären Erkrankungen. *Fortschr Neurol Psychiatr.*, **56**, 265–274.)

Muscle and neuromuscular junction

Myasthenia gravis
Eaton Lambert syndrome
Toxins (botulinum, tetanus, diphtheria)
Cholinergic crisis (overdose of anticholinesterases, insecticides)
Muscular dystrophies, myotonias
Myositides
Myopathies (toxic, endocrine)
Disorders of potassium metabolism (periodic paralyses).

Peripheral nerve

Polyneuritis (Guillain – Barré syndrome)
Polyneuropathies
Cranial nerve palsies (meningeal infiltration, Garcin syndrome, glossopharyngeal neuralgia).

Central nervous system

Ischaemias (brain stem infarction, lacunar infarcts, Binswanger's disease, multiple infarcts, pseudobulbar palsy, haemorrhages)
Craniocerebral trauma
Infratentorial tumours (cerebro-pontine angle, clivus)
Craniovertebral junction anomalies
Extrapyramidal motor disorders (Parkinsonism, Wilson's disease, chorea, dystonia, myoclonias)
Spinocerebellar diseases (Friedreich's ataxia, olivopontocerebellar degeneration)
Anterior horn cell diseases (motor neuron disease, poliomyelitis)
Inflammatory disorders (encephalitis, multiple sclerosis, syphilis, rabies).

MEMORIX NEUROLOGY

Diagnostic criteria of cranial (temporal) arteritis

1. Raised ESR (often >100 mm, mostly >50 mm/h).
2. Age >45 years.
3. Continuous head pains, often worst in temples, with touch tenderness, occasionally distended temporal arteries, aggravated by mastication ('claudication'),
   and/or
   disorders of vision, including sudden blindness which is permanent
   and/or
   arthralgia and periarticular myalgia of proximal joints (polymyalgia rheumatica), possibly polyneuropathy.

Additional features: hypochromic anaemia
raised alkaline phosphatase
raised angiotensin converting enzyme
biopsy of temporal or occipital artery (giant cell arteritis, immunological testing: deposition of immunoglobulin & complement).

Treatment: corticosteroids, equivalent to prednisolone 1 mg/kg body weight urgently, as soon as diagnosis is suspected. Long-term treatment for at least 1 year, reducing dose according to ESR and clinical response.

Laboratory investigations in suspected vasculitis and collagenoses

1. Sytemic inflammation
   ESR, C-reactive protein
   Immunoglobulins A, G, M, E
   Complement C3, C4, C9
   Full blood count (including differential WBC)
   Circulating immune complexes

2. Collagen vascular disorders
   Autoantibodies (ANA, es- + dsDNA, ENA group, SSA, SSB)
   Rheumatoid factor (Rose–Waaler)

3. Infections
   Antibodies against Borrelia, Salmonella, Yersinia
   Viral antibodies
   Syphilis serology
   Hepatitis screening
   Cryoglobulins
   Paraproteins
   CSF: cell count, total protein, IgG, IgA, IgM, oligoclonal bands

4. Visceral involvement
   Transaminases
   Creatinine clearance
   Urine: protein, casts, eosinophils

5. Associated coagulation disorders
   PT, PTT
   Antiphopholipid antibodies

6. Other
   Anticytoplasmic antineutrophil antibodies (eANCA)

   (Screening tests underlined)

MULTIFOCAL NEUROLOGICAL DISORDERS

Vasculitis survey

	CNS	PNS	Muscle	Other organ involvement	Complement level (C3, 4)	Important laboratory tests	Biopsy confirmation
Primary vasculitides							
Polyarteritis group							
Polyarteritis nodosa	30	60	50	Kidney, heart	Lowered	Circulating immune complexes, rheumatoid factor, Hbs-Ag	Muscle, nerve
Allergic granulomatosis	25	70	20	Lung	Raised	eosinophilia, IgE, circulating immune complexes	Muscle, nerve
Giant cell arteritides							
Cranial arteritis	10	30	30	Joints (polymyalgia)	Raised	ESR, alkaline phosphatase, HLA-DR3, DR4	Temporal artery
Takayasu syndrome	40	/	/	Great vessels	Normal	Possibly ESR, HLA A10, B3, MB3, DR4	Arteries
Granulomatous angiitides							
Wegener's granulomatosis	25	15	<5	Respiratory/urogenital systems	Raised	Anticytoplasmic antibody, HLA-DR2	ENT
Lymphomatoid granulomatosis	35	25	10	Lung, skin	Normal	Lymphocytosis in leucopenia	Skin, lung
Hypersensitivity angiitis (Zeek)	10	20	10	Skin, kidney, joints	Normal	Circulating immune complexes	Skin
Secondary vasculitides							
Autoimmune diseases							
Lupus erythematosus	60	10	10	Skin, joints, heart	Lowered	ANA, dsDNS-antibody HLA-B8, A15	Skin
Rheumatoid arthritis	<5	40	50	Joints	Raised	Rheumatoid factor	Joints
Scleroderma	∇	50	90	Skin, oesophagus, joints	Normal	Rheumatoid factor	Skin
Mixed connective tissue disease	∇	10	90	Joints	Lowered	ENS antibody	Pelvic rim
Sjögren's syndrome	30	10	10	Eye, ENT (sicca)	Normal	Schirmer's test	Salivary gland
Hypersensitivity angiitis (infection, paraneoplastic, drugs)	10	20		Skin, kidney, joints	Raised	Circulating immune complexes, eosinophilia, IgE, IgA	Skin
Unclassified vasculitides							
Thromboangitis obliterans	?	–	–	Peripheral vessels	Normal	Anti-elastin antibody	Temporal Artery
Moya–Moya syndrome	100	–	–	None	Normal	Circ. imm. complexes, HLA AW24, BW46, BW54	–
Sneddon's syndrome	100	–	–	Skin (livedo racemosa)	Normal	Antiphopholipid a.b.	Skin
Cogan's syndrome	?	–	–	Eye, ear	Normal	ESR, CSF, HLA BW17	Skin
Isolated CNS angiitis	100	–	–	None	Normal	–	Brain
Behçet's syndrome	30	–	–	Mucosae (aphthous ulcers), eye	C9 raised	Circ. immune complexes, CSF, HLA B5, B12, DR7	Skin

(Gordon, M. *et al*. (1993) Relapses in patients with systemic vasculitis. *Quarterly Journal of Medicine*, **86**, 779–789.)

MEMORIX NEUROLOGY

Neurological effects of vitamin deficiencies

(Reproduced after Neundörfer, B. (1990) Neurologische Störungen bei Hyper- und Hypovitaminosen. *Nervenarzt*, **51**, 207–216.)

Vitamin	Occurs in	Effect of deficiency
A	Milk, butter, cod liver oil, egg yolk, carrots, spinach	Optic atrophy (?), benign intracranial hypertension from excess
B_1	Meat, eggs, grain, rice, yeast, potato	Beriberi polyneuropathy, Wernicke's encephalopathy
Nicotinic acid	Meat, liver, milk, peas, potato, yeast	Pellagra (encephalomyelopathy, dementia, diarrhoea, dermatitis)
B_6	Meat, grain, yeast	Nitrofurantoin and INH polyneuropathy, infantile spasms. (polyneuropathy from excess)
B_{12}	Liver, pancreas, kidney	Subacute combined degeneration of cord, mental symptoms, polyneuropathy, burning feet syndrome, optic atrophy
Folic acid	Liver, kidney, leaf vegetables	Subacute combined degeneration? Polyneuropathy (with anticonvulsant treatment)
C	Citrus fruits, fresh vegetables, liver, milk, potato	Scurvy, bleeding diathesis
D	Fish, oil, egg yolk, unskimmed milk	Tetany, osteomalacia, myopathy (rickets), rarely: epileptic fits, extrapyramidal symptoms
E	Grain, soya beans	Cerebellar degeneration
K	Spinach, green vegetables	Haemorrhages from disorders of clotting

Stages of normal sleep during one night

(Reproduced after Jovanovic, U.J. *Normal Sleep in Man*, published by Hippokrates, Stuttgart, 1971.)

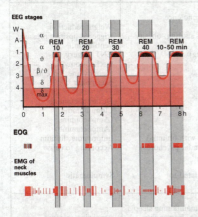

The basic sleep structure consists of **rhythms of periods of sleep** consisting of **four stages of non-REM (NREM)** and of **one stage of REM sleep**; average duration of periods 100 min, repeated 3–5 times per night.

The five stages may be defined by the **EEG**. During each period the depth of sleep increases (NREM 1–4), then lessens.

At the end of each period there is a fifth stage with rapid eye movements (**REM sleep**) which may be recorded by an electro-oculogram (EOG). **Dreams** occur particularly during REM sleep.

MEMORIX NEUROLOGY

Sleep disorders

	Treatment

Hypersomnia
 DOES: disorders of excessive somnolence
 a. Sleep apnoea syndrome
     Obstructive (90%): stentorous snoring, obesity
     (Pickwickian syndrome)
     Central (10% nocturnal waking)
	Weight reduction, triggered positive pressure ventilation, ENT surgery, tracheostomy theophylline, phrenic pacemaker

b. Narcolepsy
    Paroxysmal sleeping
    Cataplexy attacks
    Waking attacks
    Hypnagogic hallucinations
	Dexamphetamine Clomipramine (Amphetamine) (Amphetamine)

c. Kleine–Levin syndrome (men with bulimia)	Imipramine, lithium
d. Psychiatric disorders (cyclothymia, psychoses)	According to cause
e. Alcohol or drug dependency	
f. Other toxic causes	
g. Lack of sleep, hypersomnia related to menstruation	Symptomatic
Insomnia and hyposomnia DIMS: disorders of intiating and maintaining sleep a. Psychiatric diseases (cyclothymia, personality disorders)	According to cause
b. Psychosomatic hyposomnia	Symptomatic
c. Alcohol or drug dependency	Chlormethiazole, neuroleptics
d. Situational hyposomnia (extraneous disturbances)	Benzodiazepines
e. Pharmacogenic hyposomnia (after analgesics, etc.)	Thymoleptics
f. Symptomatic hyposomnia (hyperthyroidism, etc.)	According to cause
Parasomnia (motor and psychogenic sleep disorders) a. Night terrors (children)	? Tonsillectomy, benzodiazepines
b. Sleep walking (children, juveniles)	Benzodiazepines
c. Nocturnal (hypnagogic) myoclonus	Benzodiazepines
d. Enuresis (after fifth year)	Alarm device, imipramine
e. Bruxism	Benzodiazepines
f. Restless leg syndrome	Benzodiazepines, laevo-dopa
Disorders of sleep–waking cycles a. Jet lag b. Shift work c. Non-24 h sleep–waking rhythm d. Crescendo sleep–waking rhythm e. Syndrome of delayed or prolonged sleep phases	Symptomatic

MULTIFOCAL NEUROLOGICAL DISORDERS

Pathogenesis of obstructive sleep apnoea

(Reproduced after Hierholzer, K. and Schmidt, R.F. Pathophysiologie des Menschen, published by VCH, Weinheim, 1991.)

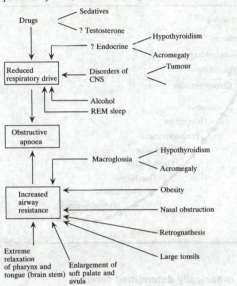

Varieties of sleep apnoea

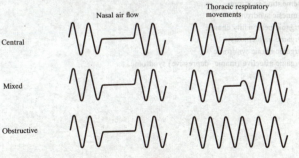

MEMORIX NEUROLOGY

Therapeutic problems in neurology
Effectiveness profile of neuroleptic drugs

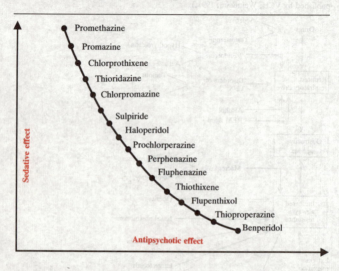

Classification of organically determined cerebral psychosyndromes (after DSM III-R)
- Delirious syndrome
- Dementing syndrome
- Amnesic syndrome
- Organic personality change
- Organic hallucinosis
- Organic manic syndrome
- Organic affective (manic–depressive) syndrome.

Treatment with botulinum toxin

(Reproduced after American Association of Neurologists (1990) The clinical usefulness of botulinum toxin. *Neurology*, **40**, 1332; Jankovic, L., Schwartz, K. and Donovan, D. (1990) *Journal of Neurology, Neurosurgery and Psychiatry*, **53**, 633–639.)

	Injection sites	BTX × (MU) USA	BTX × (ng) UK	Improvement (%)	Benefit duration (weeks)	Treatment alternatives	Side-effects
Focal dystonias Blepharospasm	Orbicularis oculi muscle (upper lid lateral and medial, lower lid lateral)	5 each	1.5 each	>90	12–15	Baclofen, clonazepam, tetrabenazine, benzhexol	Ptosis, double or blurred vision, lacrimation
Oromandibular dystonia	Jaw opening: submental muscle Jaw closing: masseters, pterygoids muscles	50 each	15 each	50–70	11	Baclofen, tetrabenazine, benzhexol	Dysphagia
Spastic dysphonia (laryngeal dystonia)	Thyroarytenoid muscles (uni- or bilaterally)	2–5	0.5–1.5	75–95	12	Speech therapy	Dysphonia, hoarseness, dysphagia
Spasmodic torticollis	Sternomastoid, trapezius latissimus dorsi muscles	50–70	15–20	60	12	Benzodiazepines, tetrabenazine	Neck weakness, dysphagia
Limb muscle dystonia	EMG guided	5–10 per muscle	1.5–3 per muscle	50–80	9	Behaviour therapy, benzhexol	Local paresis
Other movement disorders Hemifacial spasms	By clinical and EMG criteria	5 per muscle	1.5 per muscle	>90	20	Surgery, phenytoin, carbamazepine	Facial weakness
Essential tremor (head, neck, hand)	Neck or upper limb muscles	200 (neck) 15 (arms)	60 (neck) 15 (upper limb)		10	Beta-blockers, primidone	Local pareses

BTX: botulinum toxin; MU: mouse units. USA: 1 MU = 0.4 ng toxin; UK: 1 MU = 0.125 ng toxin

Neurological medication in pregnancy

Anticonvulsant treatment
If possible minimal dose monotherapy, but pregnancy may raise requirement
If possible avoid valproate in first trimester (risk of neural tube defect)
When valproate used in first trimester re-check alpha-fetoprotein, ? amniocentesis
With carbamazepine stop breast-feeding
Barbiturates and benzodiazepines are possible alternative drugs
No benzodiazepines during breast-feeding, stop if indicated
With primidone treatment use vitamin K prophylaxis in last pregnancy month (injection treatment for baby)
Prophylactic use of folic acid 2.5 mg–5 mg daily with anticonvulsants.

Analgesic treatment
During pregnancy no non-steroidal anti-inflammatory drugs or phenazone derivatives
If necessary paracetamol or aspirin (but avoid aspirin in third trimester if possible)
Strong analgesics to be avoided during breast-feeding (opioids, pentazocine)
No ergot derivatives during pregnancy
No dihydroergotamine injections during pregnancy or lactation
No serotonin antagonists (pizotifen) during pregnancy
Beta-blockers only if strongly indicated

Treatment of infections
Penicillins and cephalosporins if strongly indicated
No tetracyclines, no aminoglycosides
Nitrofurantoin, sulphonamides and chloramphenicol not suitable in third trimester and during breast-feeding
Erythromycin unsuitable during breast-feeding
Metronidazole not to be used in first trimester and during breast-feeding
Tuberculostatic treatment: use isoniazid and ethambutol
No pyrazinamide, no streptomycin
Use acyclovir only if strongly indicated (teratogenicity).

Other treatments
No immunosuppressants during pregnancy (stop azathioprine 6 months before planned pregnancy)
Anticholinesterases allowed if strongly indicated, no pyridostigmine with lactation
No nimodipine during pregnancy
No dantrolene, tizanidine during pregnancy; possible alternatives baclofen, diazepam
If possible avoid phenoxybenzamine (carbachol a possible alternative).

THERAPEUTIC PROBLEMS IN NEUROLOGY

Options for plasmapheresis treatment in neurology

	Number of treatments	Special considerations
Myasthenia gravis	6–10	Additional prednisolone, azathioprine (interval treatments)
Acute Guillain–Barré syndrome	10–15	Preliminary exclusion of causal infections; treatment start no later than 2 weeks from onset of symptoms. Evoked muscle action potentials ≤20% of normal
Paraproteinaemic polyneuropathy	6	Additional corticosteroids
Eaton Lambert syndrome	6–10	Only if severe, additional immunosuppressants (azathioprine)
Myositis	6–10	Only if life-threatening; additional cyclophosphamide and corticosteroids
Chronic relapsing polyneuropathy	5–10 (intermittently)	In case azathioprine does not control

Options for immunosuppressant treatment in neurology

Treatment mode	Effect on	Possible indications
Corticosteroids	Non-specific (inhibition of interleukin, of inflammation, lymphocytolysis)	Multiple sclerosis relapse, cranial arteritis, myositis, myasthenia gravis, paraproteinaemic polyneuropathy, chronic relapsing polyneuropathy
Azathioprine	T cells (cell-mediated immune reaction), antimetabolic (inhibitors of purine synthesis)	Myasthenia gravis, multiple sclerosis (? relapse prevention) Eaton Lambert syndrome, immunovasculitis
Cyclophosphamide	Antibody production (humoral immune reaction), alkylating substance	Immunovasculitides, multiple sclerosis, paraproteinaemic polyneuropathies
Cyclosporine A	T cells (cell-mediated immune reaction) activation inhibited	Myasthenia gravis, multiple sclerosis
Plasmapheresis	Antibody production, non-specific mediators eliminated	Guillain–Barré syndrome, chronic relapsing polyneuropathy, myasthenia gravis, myositis, Eaton Lambert syndrome (severe), paraproteinaemic polyneuropathy, acute multiple sclerosis
7S immunoglobulin	Antibody	Guillain–Barré syndrome, CIDP (chronic inflammatory demyelinating polyneuropathy), multiple sclerosis
Thymectomy	T cell production inhibited	Myasthenia gravis
Splenectomy	Reduced production of immunocompetent cells	Myasthenia gravis

Immunosuppressant treatment options in neurological diseases

(Modified after Kappos, L. (1993) Immuntherapie. *Gelbe Hefte*, **33**, 118–127.)

Diagnosis	First choice	Second choice
Neuromuscular diseases		
Myositis	Corticosteroids + azathioprine	Plasma exchange, cyclophosphamide
Myasthenia gravis	Thymectomy: azathioprine + corticosteroids	Plasma exchange
Polyneuritis		
Acute	Plasma exchange, Ig	Corticosteroids (?)
CIDP	Corticosteroids, plasma exchange	Cyclophosphamide, Ig
Monoclonal gammopathies	Corticosteroids, plasma exchange	Cyclophosphamide, Ig
Central nervous system		
Multiple sclerosis*		
Acute relapse	Corticosteroids	Cyclophosphamide ± plasma exchange
Prevention of relapses/progressive[†]	Azathioprine	CyA, cyclophosphamide, Mitox, IFNbeta, COP 1, oral MBP
Primary chronic progressive[†]	Cyclophophamide	Mitox, CyA, TLI, intrathecal steroids
ADEM	Corticosteroids	Plasma exchange, Ig, cyclophophamide
Behçet's disease	Corticosteroids, azathioprine	CyA, chlorambucil, thalidomide
Chronic meningitis	Intrathecal cytarabine	Corticosteroids
CNS-limited vasculitis	Corticosteroids + cyclophosphamide	–

Ig: intravenous immunoglobulin; CyA: cyclosporin A; Mitox: ifosfamide (alkylating cytotoxic 'Mitoxana'); IFNbeta: beta interferon; COP 1: copolymer 1; TLI: total lymphoid irradiation (as for Hodgkin's disease); CIDP: chronic inflammatory demyelinating polyneuropathy; ADEM: acute disseminated encephalomyelitis
* Ebers, G.C. (1994) Treatment of multiple sclerosis. *Lancet*, **343**, 273–279 for critical discussion
[†] no drugs have been shown definitely to slow disease progression

CHROMOSOME ANOMALIES

Chromosome anomalies in neurological diseases

Disease	Affected chromosome	DNA diagnosis availability
Alzheimer's dementia (familial form)	21 Q	No
Ataxia-telangiectasia (Louis–Bar)	11 Q 23	Limited
Autosomal recessive muscular dystrophies	6	No
Benign familial seizures	20 Q	No
Central core disease	19 Q 12	No
Charcot–Marie–Tooth disease	1 Q 21; 17 Q 11	No
Chronic muscular dystrophies of childhood	5 Q	No
Duchenne/Becker muscular dystrophies	Xp 21 (dystrophin)	Yes
Dystrophia myotonica	19 Q 13	Yes
Emery–Dreifuss muscular dystrophy	Xq 28	Yes
Familial amyloid neuropathy	18 Q	No
Facioscapulohumeral muscular dystrophy	4 Q 31	No
Friedreich's ataxia	9 Q 13–21	Yes
Gaucher's disease	1 Q 21	Limited
Huntington's disease	4 P 16	Yes
Hyperkalaemic familial paralysis	17 Q 31	Limited
Kugelberg–Welander muscular atrophy	5 Q	Limited
Meningioma	14	No
Neurofibromatosis I (Recklinghausen)	17 Q 11	Yes
Neurofibromatosis II (acoustic neuroma)	22 Q 11	Limited
Paramyotonia congenita	17 Q 31	Limited
Spinocerebellar degeneration	6 P 21	No
Torsion dystonia	9 Q 34	Limited
Tuberous sclerosis	9 Q, 11 Q, 12 Q	Limited
Von Hippel–Lindau disease	3 P 25	Limited
Werdnig–Hoffmann disease	5 Q 11	Limited
Wilson's disease	13 Q 14	Limited

INDEX

Index

Acalculia 51
ACTH 130
Adenohypophyseal hormones 130
Adrenal cortex disorders, neurological features 252
Adrenal medulla disorders, neurological features 252
Agnosia, object 51
Agraphia 51
Aids
  dementia complex (ADC), stages 172
  neurological complications 171–2
  opportunistic infections 171
  see also HIV infection
Alcoholism
  AEPs 84
  nervous system/muscle disorders 258
Alcohol withdrawal, management 259
Alexia 51
Alzeimer type dementia
  biochemical/structural abnormalities 147
  definition 147
  differential diagnosis 147
  prevalence 147
Amblyopia, tobacco–alcohol 258
Amino acid metabolism, disorders 144
Amnesia 51
Amyloid neuopathies, hereditary 214
Anaesthesia dolorosa 31
Analgesics, and pregnancy 268
Angiomatosis, racemose, intracerebral 256
Anhidrosis 42, 43
Anisocoria, clinical/pharmacological differentiation 6
Anosognosia, grades 51
Anterior communicating artery 175
Antibiotics
  brain abscesses 165
  CSF entry 166
  in neurological infections 165, 166
Anticholinesterases, dosages, in myasthenia 248
Anticoagulants 103
  in acute cerebral infarction 183
Anticonvulsants
  choice, and epilepsy type 157
  doses/pharmacology 158
  and pregnancy 268

reactions/side-effects/overdosage features 159
Antidiuretic hormone (ADH) 129
Aphasia 51
  types 52
Apnoea 56
Apomorphine test, in Parkinsonism 207
Apraxia 51
Argyll Robertson pupil 5
Arnold–Chiari malformation, types 208
Ataxias 143
Ataxia telangiectasia 256
Atropine effect 5
Attacks
  non-epileptic 162
  see also Collapse, sudden, diagnosis; Epilepsy; Fits
Auditory evoked potentials (AEPs)
  diagnostic criteria 81
  diagnostic indications 82
  normal values 85
  peak drop-out, and lesion site 81
  in various diseases 84
Auditory pathways, AEP origin sites 83
Auerbach's (myenteric) plexus 41
Autonomic nervous system 41–9
  function assessment 44

Barthel scale 186
Basal cell naevoid syndrome 256
Basal ganglia, functions 131
Bimastoid line, craniovertebral junction 109
Biot's respiration 56
Bladder
  disorders 46–9
  neuroanatomy 48
  see also Neurogenic bladder disorders
  function 46
  musculature 46
Blink reflex, EMG normal range 78
Blood clotting
  factors 103
  tests 103
Blood supply, cerebral
  arterial
    anatomy 112
    carotid system 112
    collaterals 175
    extracranial, arteriosclerosis

INDEX

frequency 179
 sonography 63, 65, 66
 vascular territories 181
 vertebro-basilar system 112
 venous drainage, anatomy 188
Botulinum toxin, in treatment 267
Bournville's syndrome 256
Brachial plexus lesions 224, 225, 235
 differences from cervical root lesions 223
Brachial plexus, spinal root supply, peripheral distribution 225
Brain
 abscesses, causative organisms/ antibiotic therapy 165
 herniation and raised ICP 124
 mapping, EEG 72
 syndromes 61–2
 tumours
  localization 121, 123
  radiotherapy/cytostatic therapy indications 122
  treatment and follow-up 121–2
Brain death 129
 criteria 203–4
Brainstem
 crossed syndromes 180
 vascular syndromes, AEPs 84
Branching enzyme deficiency 239

C7 root syndrome 236
C8 root syndrome 235
CAMBS scale, multiple sclerosis 254
Carbohydrate disorders 144
Carotid stenosis, Doppler sonography 66
Carpal tunnel syndrome 236
Cartography, brain, EEG 72
Cauda equina syndrome 204
Causalgia 31
Central nervous system, integrative functions 50
Cerebellar degeneration 258
 acquired 145
 congenital 143
 and infections 145
 metabolic 145
 paraneoplastic 145
 toxic 145
Cerebellum 40
 afferent and efferent pathways 38
 hemispheres, and motor function 38–9
 pars intermedia, and motor function 38
 vermis, and motor function 38

Cerebral aneurysms
 neurological defects after 191
 sites 191
Cerebral arteries, vascular territories 181
Cerebral cortex
 integrative functions 50
 left hemisphere 50
 magnetic stimulation 96
Cerebral functions, disorders 39
Cerebral hemispheres, cognitive differences, dextrad persons 54
Cerebral infarction, *see* Infarction, cerebral
Cerebral ischaemia, *see* Ischaemia, cerebral
Cerebral venous drainage, anatomy 188
Cerebral venous sinus thrombosis
 causes/associated disorders 189
 symptoms and signs 189
Cerebrospinal fluid (CSF) 97
 abnormalities 98
  cerebrovascular disease 101
  myopathies 102
  nervous system diseases 99–100
  in polyneuropathies 102
 antibiotic entry 166
 and infections, immunological tests 102
Cerebrovascular accidents
 independence after, assessment scale 187
 localization 177
 see also Stroke
Cerebrovascular diseases 173–95
 CSF changes 101
Cerebrovascular territories, CT 179
Cervical spine root lesions, intervertebral disc prolapse 220
Chamberlain's line, craniovertebral junction 109
Cheyne–Stokes respiration 56
Chinizarin (starch) test, for sweating 45
Cholinergic crisis, differences from myasthenic crisis 249
Chorea
 aetiology and treatment 139
 types 139
Choroidal arteries 175
Chromosomes, anomalies, in neurological diseases 271
Claude syndrome 200
Claw hand 227
Cluster headache, chronic paroxysmal hemicrania differentiation 117

MEMORIX NEUROLOGY

Collagenoses, laboratory investigations 260
Collapse, sudden, diagnosis 160–1
Common peroneal nerve
  conduction velocities 76
  distal latencies and age 76
  lesions 229
Compartment syndromes 231
Computerized tomography (CT)
  cerebrovascular territories 177
  changes in cerebral infarction 176
  contrast injection, brain lesions 111
  skull 110–11
Confusional states, differential diagnosis 150
Consciousness, disorders, causes 58
Conus medullaris syndrome 205
Corpus callosum anastomoses 175
Cortical dementia, differences from subcortical dementia 149
Cranial nerves
  function/testing 2–3
  lesions
    causes 2–3
    and eye movements 8
    nerve III, and light reaction 5
  multiple deficits, differential diagnosis 20
  trauma 199
Cranial (temporal) arteritis, diagnostic criteria 260
Craniocerebral trauma
  AEPs 84
  anticonvulsant prophylaxis 200
  clinical grading 195
  clinical stages 197–8
  and epilepsy 200
    frequency 200
  Glasgow Coma Scale 196
  Glasgow Outcome Scale 196
  surgery indications 195
Craniovertebral junction, X-ray assessment measurements 109
Crossed brainstem syndromes 180
Cutaneous reflexes, peripheral nerves/spinal roots 24
Cytostatic chemotherapy, indications, in brain tumours 122

Deafness
  causes 16
  conductive 16
  end-organ (cochlear), AEPs 84
  perceptive 16
Delerium tremens 258
Dementia
  and AIDS 172
  cortical/subcortical, differential diagnosis 149
  differential diagnosis 146
  vascular, diagnosis 148
  see also individual types
Denervation, EMG findings 73
Dermatomes, peripheral sensory nerves 33–4
Detrusor
  areflexia 46
  hyperreflexia 46
  sphincter dyssynergia 46
Diabetic amyotrophy 234
Digastric line, craniovertebral junction 109
Disorientation in space 51
Dizziness
  causes 19
  differential diagnosis 19
Doppler sonography 63–6
  carotid stenosis 66
  transcranial 64
    intracranial arteries indentification 65
Dorsal interosseus muscle, magnetic stimulation 96
Dysaesthesia 31
Dysarthrias, neurological 55
Dyskalaemic periodic paralyses 251
Dyskinesia 140
Dystonia 140

Elderly, confusional states, differential diagnosis 150
Electroencephalography (EEG) 67–72
  cartography 72
  diagnostic criteria 67
  electrode positioning, in 10–20 system 68
  frequency bands 69
  normal variants 70
  rhythms, statistical distribution 69
  sleep stages 71
Electromyography (EMG) 73–8
  F wave/H reflex/blink reflex, normal range 78
  individual muscles, normal findings 74
  normal findings 73, 74
  patterns 73–4

INDEX

procedures 73
repetitive nerve stimulation 78
Encephalitis
  herpes simplex 163
  viral 163
    differential diagnosis 164
Endarterectomy, internal carotid, indications 184
Endocrine disorders
  and attacks 162
  neurological features 252
Epiconus syndrome 205
Epilepsia partialis continua, childhood 152, 153
Epilepsy
  acute, treatment 153
  age-related, classification 152
  central threshold, lowering by drugs 151
  and craniocerebral trauma 200
  first aid 154
  international classification 151–3
  non-age-related, classification 152
  prognosis 154
  psychomotor, treatment 153
  types, anti-epileptic drug choice 157
  see also Grand mal; Petit mal, treatment; Status epilepticus
Evoked potentials
  latency ranges 79
  see also various types
Eye movements
  in cranial nerve lesions 8
  and visual field defects 10–11

Face and head neuralgias
  drug therapy 120
  pain localization 118–19
  types 119
Facial palsies
  causes 13
  lesion levels 14
Femoral nerve, lesions 230, 234
Ferguson reflex 129
Fibrinolytic agents 103
Fist, posture making 226
Fits 151–9
  causes, and age 153
  see also Attacks; Epilepsy
Follicle-stimulating hormone (FSH) 130
Forbes' disease 239
Foville syndrome 180
FTA–ABS 168

F wave, EMG normal range 78

Gasparini syndrome 180
Gasping 56
Glasgow Coma Scale 196
Glasgow Outcome Scale 196
Gluteal nerve, lesions 230
Glycogenoses 239
Gorlin–Goltz syndrome 256
Grand mal
  differential diagnosis 156
  treatment 153
Guillain–Barré syndrome, diagnostic criteria 215

H wave, EMG normal range 78
Haematomas, intracerebral 192–43, 197–8
Hallucinosis, alcoholic 258
Headache
  differential diagnosis 116–17
  drug-induced
    diagnostic criteria 117
    various drugs 117
  WHO classification 114–15
Hemianhidrosis 42, 43
Hemianopia
  bitemporal 10
  homonymous 10
Hemicrania, paroxysmal, chronic, cluster headache differentiation 117
Hemiplegia, cruciate 180
Herpes simplex encephalitis 162
HIV infection
  CDC classification 170
  stages 168
  Walter Reed Hospital staging 170
  see also AIDS
Holmes–Adie (myotonic) pupil 5
Horner's syndrome
  causes 7
  sweating preservation 42
Hounsfield units, CT, skull tissue density 110
Hydrocephalus, differential diagnosis 127
Hyperpathia 31
Hyperpyrexia, malignant 241
Hyperventilation, central 56
Hypothalamus
  disorders, neurological features 252
  regulatory hormones 133

Iliopsoas muscle, paralysis 230
Immunological function, disorders 144

Immunoneuropathies, varieties 216
Immunosuppressant treatment, in
 neurology 268, 269–70
Infarction, cerebral
 acute, anticoagulation 183
 clinical findings 174, 177
 concomitant diseases 173
 CT changes pattern 176
 diagnosis 174
 laboratory tests 174
 management principles 183
 neurological deficits, quantification
  scale 186
 risk factors 173
 see also Cerebrovascular accidents;
  Stroke
Infections, treatment, and pregnancy 268
Inflammatory disease, nervous system
 163–72
Internal carotid endarterectomy,
 indications 184
Intervertebral disc prolapse
 cervical spine root lesions 220
 lumbosacral spinal root lesions 221
Intracerebral haematomas
 cerebral ischaemia differentiation 192
 clinical features 194
 frequency and causes, various sites 193
 MRI 192
Intracranial arteries, sonographic
 identification 65
Intracranial bleeding
 spontaneous, diagnostic procedures 193
 traumatic 195
Intracranial pressure, raised, brain
 herniation 124
Ion channel disorders, muscular 246
Ischaemia, cerebral
 classification 173
 differences from intracerebral
  haematomas 192
 differential diagnosis 182
 index, in dementia 148

Jackson syndrome 180

Karnofsky scale, neoplasia, disability
 grading 122
Kierns–Sayre syndrome (KSS) 244
Korsakow's psychosis 258
Kurtzke impairment scale, multiple
 sclerosis 253

L4 root syndrome 234
L5 root syndrome 232
Lacunar infarcts, localization, and clinical
 syndrome 178
Lambert and Eaton myasthenic syndrome,
 electromyography 78
Language testing 53
Lateral cutaneous nerve, thigh, lesions
 230
Leber's hereditary optic neuropathy 243
Leptomeningeal anastomoses 175
LHNO 243
Limbic association cortex, integrative
 functions 50
Limb muscles
 lower, innervation 27
 upper, innervation 27
Lipid disorders 142
Lipid metabolism, disorders, neuropathies
 214
Locked-in syndrome, patient contact
 inability 201
Louis–Bar's syndrome 256
Lower limb
 muscle innervation 27
 non-radicular pain, neurological causes
  222
Lumber puncture
 CSF appearance 97
 indications 97
Lumbosacral spinal root lesions
 causes 222
 intervertebral disc prolapse 221
Luteinizing hormone (LH) 130

McArdle's disease 239
McGregor's line, craniovertebral junction
 109
McRae's line, craniovertebral junction
 109
Magnetic resonance imaging (MRI)
 and intracerebral haematomas,
  methaemoglobin 190
 planes 113
 tissue relaxation times 113
Magnetic stimulation
 motor evoked potentials (MEPs) 94
 normal ranges 96
 sites 95
Malignant hyperpyrexia 241
Marchiavafa–Bignami syndrome 258
Medial longitudinal bundle, lesions 9

INDEX

Median nerve
  conduction velocities 75
  distal latencies and age 75
  lesions 236
  palsy, causes 226
  somatosensory evoked potentials (SSEPs) 92
Meissner's (submucus) plexus 41
MELAS 243
Memory tests 53
Meningeal stretch signs 35
Meningitis
  bacterial, causative organisms/treatment 165
  chronic, causes 172
Meningocoele 207
Meningomyelocoele 207
Mental arithmetic tests 53
Mental disorders 59
  acute 60
  chronic 60
  organic 60
Mental state, assessment 59
MERFF 243
Metabolic diseases, myopathic syndromes 238
Methaemoglobin, and intracerebral haematomas 192
Micturition centres 46
Migraine, therapy 120
Millard–Gubler syndrome 180
Mitochondrial multisystem disorders, and mitochondrial DNA mutations 243–4
Mitochondrial myopathies 240
Motor conduction velocities, of nerves 75–7
Motor cortical areas, somatotropic arrangement 28
Motor disorders, of CNS 131
Motor evoked potentials (MEPs), magnetic stimulation 94
Motor functions, and cerebellum 38–9
Motor neuromuscular end-plate 247
Motor pathways 21
Motor system
  functional anatomy 23
  structure/performance/role 22
Multifocal neurological disorders 251
Multiple sclerosis
  AEPs 84
  CAMBS scale 254

classification 253
impairment (Kurtzke) scale 253
typical features 255
Multisystem degenerations 206
Muscle diseases 237–50
  CSF changes 102
  diagnostic procedures 237
  see also Myopathies
Muscles
  electrical membrane stability disorders 246
  limbs, innervation 27
  strength testing, power grades 24
  stretch reflexes, peripheral nerves/spinal roots 24
Muscular dystrophies, genetics and course 242
Mutism, akinetic, patient contact inability 201
Myasthenia, electromyography, repetitive nerve stimulation 78
Myasthenia gravis
  anticholinesterases, dosages 248
  contraindicated drugs, and alternatives 250
  grading 247
  tensilon test 248
Myasthenic crisis, differences from cholinergic crisis 249
Myelinolysis, central pontine 258
  AEPs 84
Myencephalopathies 243–4
Myoclonus
  treatment 142
  types 141
Myoglobinuria, causes 246
Myography, needle electrode 73
Myopathies
  alcoholic 258
  congenital 238–9
    benign 237
  EMG findings 74
  and metabolic diseases 238
  metabolic function tests 245
  mitochondrial 240
Myotonias, congenital 238

NARP 243
National Institutes of Health (NIH), USA, stroke scale 186
Neglect syndrome 51
Neocerebellum; function disorders 39

MEMORIX NEUROLOGY

Nerve conduction velocities 75–7
Nervous system diseases
  and attacks 162
  CSF changes 99–100
Nervous system, traumatic lesions 195–201
Nervous system tumours 121–6
  histological classification 125–6
  localization 121
Neuralgias 31
  face and head, pain localization 118–19
Neurinoma, acoustic, AEPs 84
Neurofibromatosis 256
  acoustic, bilateral 256
Neurogenic bladder disorders
  causes/treatment 49
  investigation/management 47
  lesion sites 49
Neurohypophyseal hormones 129
Neuroleptic drugs, effectiveness profile 266
Neuropsychological disorders 51
Neuropsychological tests
  bedside 53
  minimal scoring 53
Neurosyphilis
  diagnostic testing 168
  stages/clinical features 169
  treatment indications 167
Ninhydrin test, for sweating 45
Nystagmus
  differential diagnosis 17–18
  disassociated (ataxic) 9
  types 17–18
Obturator nerve, lesions 230
Occipital artery 173
Ondine's curse 56
One and half syndrome 9
Ophthalmic surgery 173
Ophthalmoplegia
  external, progressive (PEO) 244
  internuclear 9
Opportunistic infections, AIDS 171
Optic nerve lesions, and light reaction 5
Oxytocin 129

Pain
  localization, face and head neuralgias 118–19
  non-radicular, lower limb, neurological causes 222
  phantom 31
  referred, areas (Henry Head) 219
  segmental 31

Pancreas disorders, neurological features 252
Papillary light reaction 4–5
  abnormal 5
  absent/lost 5
Papilloedema
  differential diagnosis 1
  neurological symptoms 1
  neurological syndromes 1
Paraesthesia 31
Paraneoplastic neurological disorders 251
Parasympathetic nervous system 41
  functions 42, 43
Parathyroid disorders, neurological features 252
Parietotemporal association cortex, integrative functions 50
Parkinsonism
  apomorphine test 133
  causes 134
  disability grading 132
  disease staging 131
  glossary 132
  idiopathic (Parkinson's disease), diagnostic criteria 133
  treatment 136
  types 134
  see also Tremor
Parkinsonism-like syndromes 134
Peripheral nerve lesions 219–36
  causes 226–30
  classification 223
  differential diagnosis 232–6
Peripheral nerves
  and reflexes 24, 25–6
  sensory, dermatomes 33–4
Peroneal nerve, lesions 229, 232
Persistent vegetative state, patient contact inability 201
Petit mal, treatment 153
Phacomatoses 256
Phantom pain 31
Phytanic acid storage (Refsum's) disease, diet 216
Pituitary hormones
  anterior lobe 130
  posterior lobe 129
Pituitary disorders, neurological features 252
Pituitary tumours
  diagnosis 128
  symptoms and signs 128
Plasmapheresis, in neurology 269, 270

INDEX

Poisoning, CSF changes 102
Polygraph recording, physical parameters 69
Polyneuritis
  aetiology 211
  inflammatory demyelinating, chronic (CDP) 215
Polyneuropathies 210–18, 258
  aetiology 211
  autonomic involvement
    causative diseases 217
    diagnostic tests 217
    features 217
  causes
    in neurology 210, 217
    treatment 218
  CSF changes 102
  diagnostic strategies 210
  drugs and medications-associated 212
  hereditary 213
    metabolic 214
  toxic 212
Porphyrias 257
  contraindicated drugs and alternatives 257
  hereditary 214
Posterior communicating artery 175
Praxis testing 53
Prefrontal association cortex, integrative functions 50
Pregnancy, and neurological medication 268
Protoporphyria, erythropoietic 257
Pseudoptosis, causes 7
Psychic functions, range/disorders 59
Psychogenic attack, differential diagnosis 156
Psychosyndromes, cerebral, organic 266
Ptosis, causes 7
Pudendal nerve, lesions 230
Pyramidal tract, signs 36

Radial nerve
  lesions 228
  palsy, causes 228
Radiotherapy, indications, in brain tumours 122
Raymond–Céstan syndrome 180
Referred pain, areas (Henry Head) 219
Reflexes
  pathological
    manouevres 37
    significance 37

  peripheral nerves 24
    relationship 25–6
  spinal roots 24
Refsum's disease, diet 216
Respiration
  central disorders 56
  neuromuscular disorders 57
Rinne's hearing test 15

S1 root syndrome 233
Sacral plexus lesions 233
Saphenous nerve, lesions 230
Sciatic nerve, lesions 230, 232
Sensitivity, somatovisceral 29
Sensors, types 29
Sensory connections, and staging points 30, 31
Sensory cortical areas, somatotropic arrangement 28
Sensory disorders, lesion locations 29
Sensory nerves, peripheral, dermatomes 33–4
Signs, pathological 37
Skull
  calcification, and CT 111
  computerized tomography (CT) 110–11
  lesion density, CT 102–3
  X-ray, normal 104–6
Sleep
  disorders 264
  rhythm disorders, and attacks 162
  stages 263
    EEG 71
Sleep apnoea
  obstructive, pathogenesis 265
  varieties 265
Somatosensory evoked potential (SSEPs)
  abnormalities, various diseases 90
  clinical applications 89
  in diagnosis
    assessment criteria 88
    clinical significance 89
    critical data 88
    stimulation/recording sites 87
  dynamic (serial) applications 89
  lead positions 86–7
  median nerve 92
  pathophysiology 88
  prognostic significance, cerebral disorders 90
  tibial nerve 93
  trigeminal nerve 93

Somatovisceral sensitivity 29
Sonography, Doppler 63–6
Speech
  cortical area involvement 52
  disorders 51, 52, 55
Spina bifida occulta 207
Spinal cord
  anatomical levels 32
  blood supply 207
  disorders 202–9
    anatomical patterns 205
    SSEPs 91
    synopsis 209
  segments, and reflexes 25–6
  transection 203
    levels/orthotic measures 204
  transverse lesions, non-traumatic 206
  tumours, localization 121
Spinal dysraphism 207
Spinal muscular atrophies 209
Spinal roots
  anatomical levels 32
  cervical lesions, brachial plexus lesions differentiation 223
  cutaneous reflexes 24
  stretch signs 35
Spine
  vertebrae, X-rays 108
  X-rays, assessment principles 107–8
Spinocerebellar degeneration, AEPs 84
Spinocerebellar disorders
  biochemical genetics 144
  functional 39
Status epilepticus
  causes 155
  treatment 153, 157
Stretch signs, spinal roots/meningeal 35
Stroke
  differential diagnosis 182
  scale, NIH (USA) 186
  see also Cerebrovascular accidents; Infarction, cerebral; Ischaemia, cerebral
Subarachnoid haemorrhage
  early/late surgery preconditions 190
  grading 190
Subclavian steal syndrome 185
Subcortical dementia, differences from cortical dementia 149
Sudden collapse, diagnosis 160–1
Sural nerve, conduction velocities 76
Swallowing disorders, neurological causes 259

Sweating
  disorders, localization 42, 43
  pharmacological 45
  tests 45
  thermoregulatory 45
Sympathetic nervous system 41
  functions 42, 43
Sympathetic skin response (SSR) 44
Syncope 162
  differential diagnosis 156

Taste disorders, types and causes 12
Tensilon test, myasthenia gravis 248
Thalamic infarcts, blood supply/clinical features 178
Therapeutic problems 266–70
Thyroid disorders, neurological features 252
Thyroid-stimulating hormone (TSH) 130
Tibial nerve
  conduction velocities 75
  distal latencies and age 75
  lesions 229, 232
  somatosensory evoked potentials (SSEPs) 93
Tibialis
  anterior
    magnetic stimulation 96
    syndrome 231
  posterior syndrome 231
Tinnitus, causes 16
TPHA 168
Tremor
  differential diagnosis 137
  production mechanisms 138
  symptomatic, causes 137
  see also Parkinsonism
Treponema pallidum, tests for neurosyphilis 168
Triceps muscle, paralysis 228
Trigeminal nerve, somatosensory evoked potentials (SSEPs) 93
Tuberous sclerosis 256
Tumour markers, CSF 102

Ulnar nerve
  distal latencies and age 77
  lesions 235
  motor conduction velocities 77
  palsy, causes 227
Upper limb, muscle innervation 27
Urine retaining musculature 46

INDEX

Vascular dementia
  diagnosis 148
  ischaemia index 148
Vasculitis
  laboratory investigations 260, 261
  types 261
VDRL test 168
Vertebrae, anatomical levels 32
Vertigo/dizziness
  causes 19
  differential diagnosis 19
Vestibulocerebellum, function disorders 39
Visual evoked potentials (VEPs)
  abnormalities, diagnostic significance 80
  in various disorders 80
Visual field defects
  and eye movements 10–11
  lesion localization 10
  right eye/left eye 11

Visuospatial tests 53
Vitamin deficiencies
  CSF changes 102
  neurological effects 262
Volkmann's ischaemic contracture 231
von Hippel–Lindau disease 256
von Recklinghausen's disease 256

Wakefulness, disorders, and attacks 162
Wallenberg syndrome 180
Weber's hearing test 15
Weber's syndrome 180
Wernicke's encephalopathy 258
  AEPs 84
Wilson's disease, CSF tests 102
Wyburn–Mason's syndrome 256

X-rays
  skull, normal 104–6
  spinal, assessment priciples 107–8